Sylvanus Stall

What a young boy ought to know

Sylvanus Stall

What a young boy ought to know

ISBN/EAN: 9783741155376

Manufactured in Europe, USA, Canada, Australia, Japa

Cover: Foto ©Andreas Hilbeck / pixelio.de

Manufactured and distributed by brebook publishing software
(www.brebook.com)

Sylvanus Stall

What a young boy ought to know

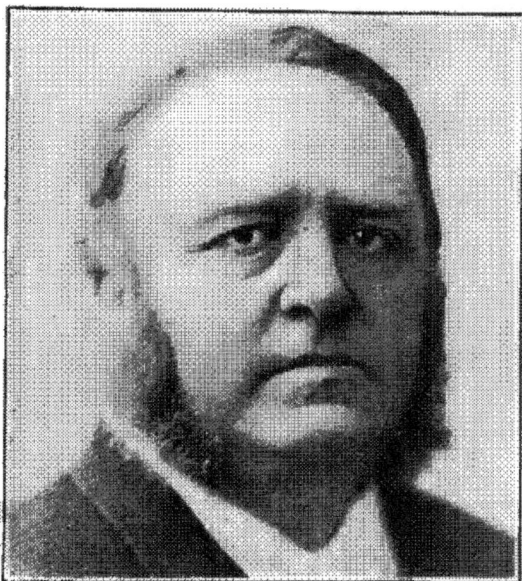

JOSEPH COOK, D.D., LL.D.

The Eminent Scholar; Boston Monday Lecturer;
author of " Biology," " Marriage," " Labor,"
" Socialism," " Occident," " Orient," etc.

" Your book on ' What a Young Boy Ought to
Know ' treats its subject with the utmost delicacy
and lucidity and is severely faithful in its admonitions
to parents as well as to the young. It is everywhere
suggestive, inspiring, and strategic in a degree, as I
think, not hitherto matched in literature of its class.
Its wide circulation ought to fall on the hearts of the
young in their thrifty and jubilant vernal season as a
divine benediction of light and heat and rain."

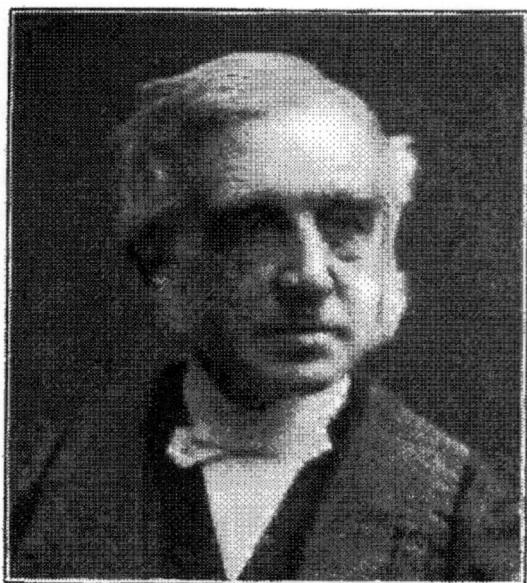

THEODORE L. CUYLER, D.D.

The best living writer of devotional literature; former pastor of Lafayette Avenue Church, Brooklyn; author of "Christianity in the Home," "How to be a Pastor," "Stirring the Eagle's Nest," "Young Preacher," etc.

"Your *admirable* little book, 'What a Young Boy Ought to Know,' ought to be in every home where there is a boy. You deserve the thanks of every parent in the land."

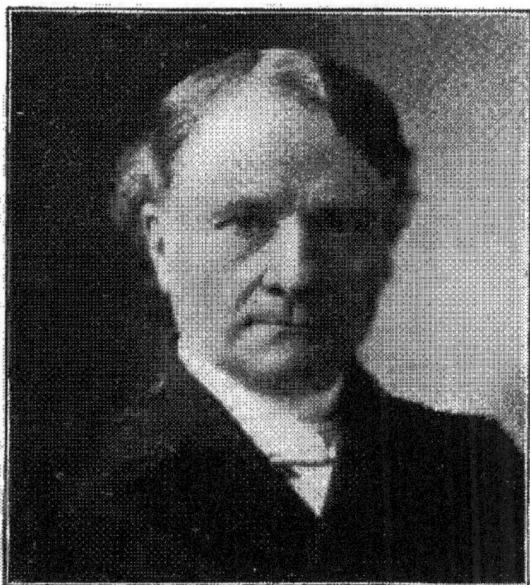

CHARLES L. THOMPSON, D.D.

Pastor of the Madison Avenue Presbyterian Church, New
York City; ex-Moderator of the General Assembly
of the Presbyterian Church; President of the
Open and Institutional Church League;
Associate Editor of *The Open
Church Magazine*, etc.

"I want to tell you how much I appreciate your
little book. It is indeed what boys ought to know
—the failure to know which has been the cause of
many sorrows and pains and penalties. Why was
not this book written centuries ago? How prudish
and false to human interests is the feeling which has
kept this knowledge back. You have presented it
with admirable delicacy and fidelity, and for one I
thank you for it."

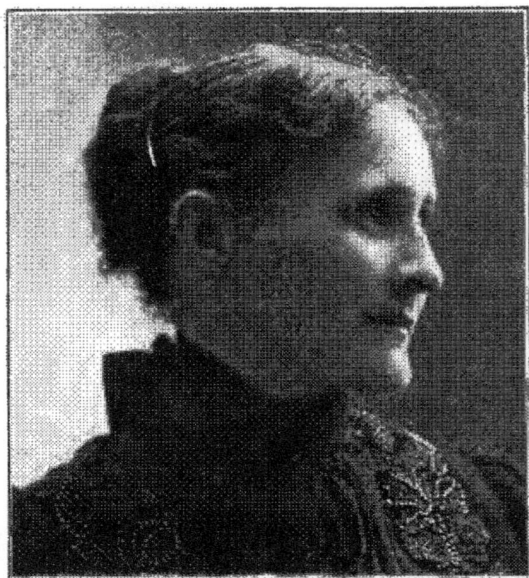

MRS. KATE WALLER BARRETT, M.D., D.Sc.
National Superintendent of the Florence Crittenton
Missions.

" If every mother and father in the world could be
made to read Dr. Stall's book, and to enter into the
spirit of it, it would do more to promote the cause of
right living than anything I know. I have been studying methods and means, looking to the bringing about
of such an understanding of the sex question as is por-
trayed in Dr. Stall's book, for the past twenty-one
years, and I unhesitatingly say that he seems to me
to have gotten more nearly to the object aimed at,
which is to make a boy feel the responsibility of the
potentiality of the father within him than any other
person I know ; the most delicate points of sex relations are handled in a manner clear, concise, and without one word to awaken morbid sentiment.   ' What a
Young Boy Ought to Know ' is verily scientific, and
yet is as readable as a fairy story.   No home is complete without it."

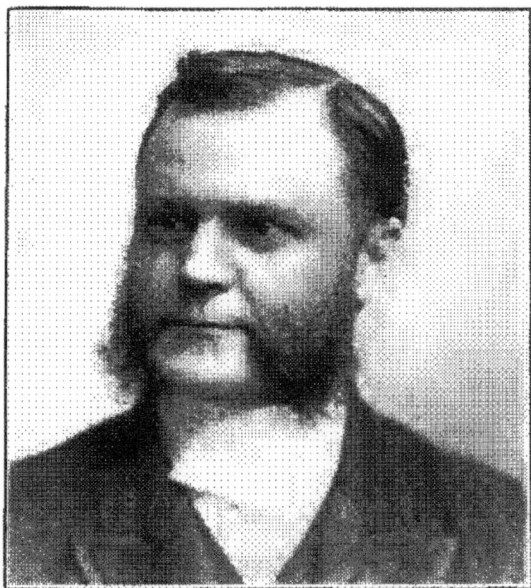

J. A. WORDEN, D.D.

The Eminent Sunday-School Worker.

" Your book, ' What a Young Boy Ought to Know,'
must have been given unto you by the Father in
heaven, both in its conception and composition. The
idea of cleansing the heart and way of the young
man by God's truth in His works as well as in His
word is a suggestion of the Spirit. Your manner of
elucidating and elaborating these facts and truths is in
the first place *faithful*, then *delicate*, and avoids both
coarseness and prudishness. May God bless and use
your book which He has evidently animated."

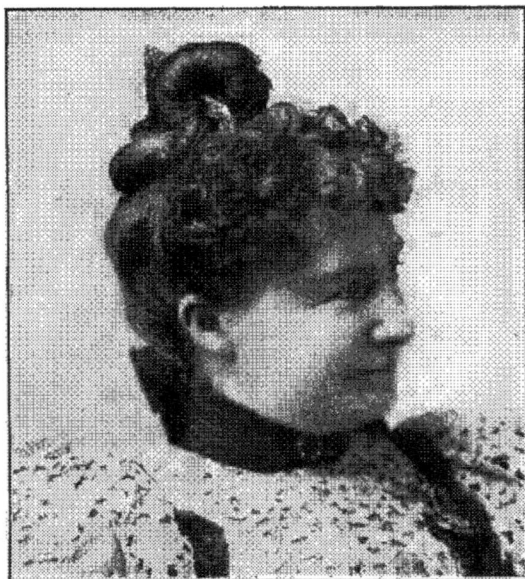

MRS. ALICE LEE MOQUÉ.

Author of " Woman : Her Heart, Soul, and Body ;"
journalist and philanthropist.

" As a woman, working with hand and brain for the
purity and uplifting of both sexes, I thank you for your
noble little book, ' What a Young Boy Ought to Know,'
—as a mother, with three growing boys of my own,
resting on my heart, I bless you for your brave words
of warning and pray that the good seeds planted may
take root in the hearts of all your youthful readers.
Ignorance is a deadly sin. In this enlightened age we
must recognize that ignorance is not innocence and
remember that to forewarn our boys is to forearm them.
The truth properly told has never yet harmed a child ;
silence, false shame, and mystery have corrupted the
souls and bodies of untold millions."

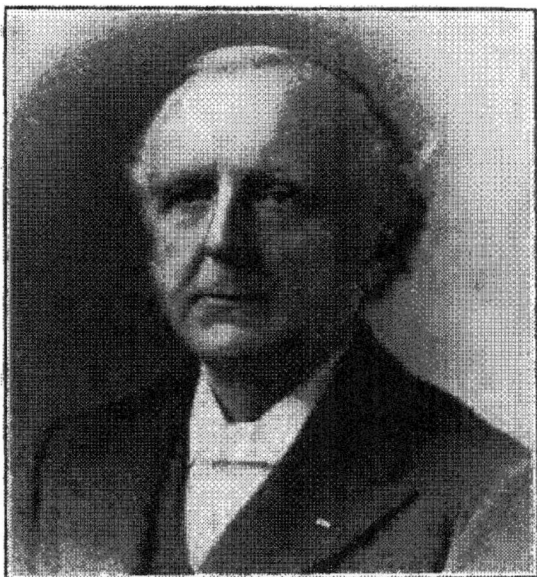

REV. F. B. MEYER, B.A.

Minister of Christ Church, Westminster, London ; author
of " Israel, A Prince with God," " Elijah ; Tried
by Fire," " The Bells of Is," etc., etc.

"The questions which are dealt with in the ' Self
and Sex Series' of books are always being asked,
and if the answer is not forthcoming from pure and
wise lips it will be obtained through vicious and em-
pirical channels. I therefore greatly commend this
series of manuals, which are written lucidly and
purely, and will afford the necessary information without pandering to unholy and sensual passion. There
has been, in my judgment, too much reticence on the
whole of this subject, and nameless sins have origi-
nated in ignorance or in the directions given to young
life by vicious men. I should like to see a wide and
judicious distribution of this literature among Christian circles."

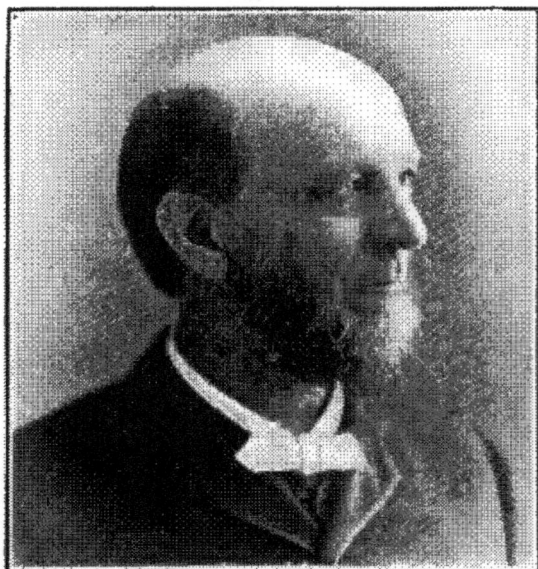

BISHOP JOHN H. VINCENT, D.D., LL.D.

Chancellor of Chautauqua University; author of "Sunday
School Institutes and Normal Classes," "The
Church School and its Officers," etc.

"You have handled with great delicacy and wisdom an exceedingly difficult subject; one which it
is almost dangerous to broach, but which *must* be
presented to the growing boy and to his parents in
a frank way, and with forcible, practical, scientific
hints for prevention and correction. Your work has
been well done."

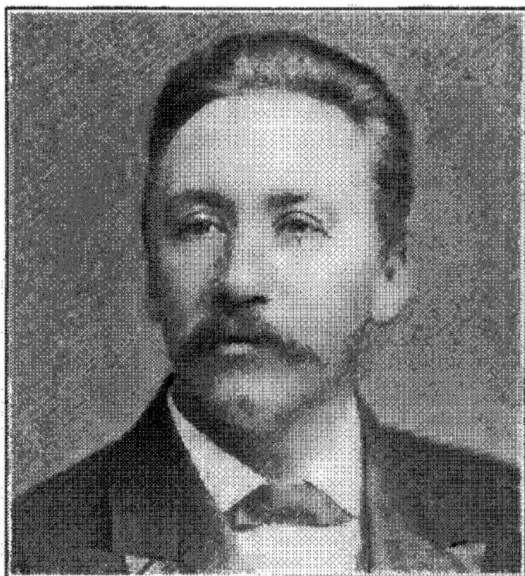

REV. THOMAS SPURGEON.

Pastor of Metropolitan Tabernacle, President of
Pastor's College, Author "The Gospel of
Grace of God," "Scarlet Thread and
Bits of Blue," "Down to the
Sea," etc.

"If it is deemed advisable to put such
information into the hands of boys I cannot
imagine it possible to have it in better form
than in 'What a Young Boy Ought to
Know.'"

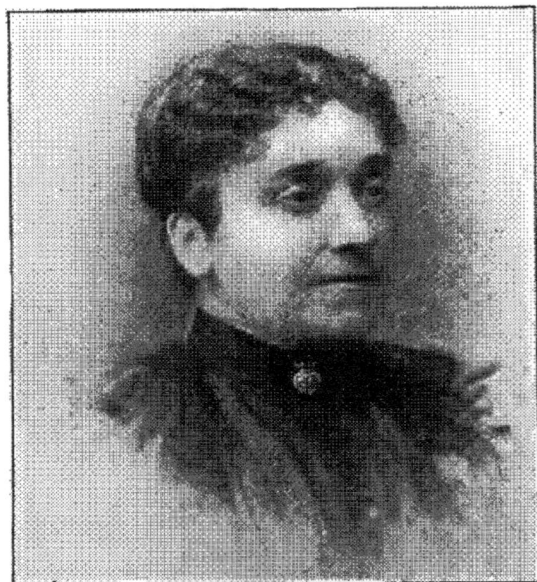

LADY HENRY SOMERSET.

Philanthropist, President National British Temperance Association, President World's Christian Temperance Union, established and edited "Woman's Signal," etc.

"I think 'What a Young Boy Ought to Know' is calculated to do an immense amount of good. I sincerely hope it may find its way to many homes in which it may be a blessing. I have long felt that we do not do enough to warn our children against the particular difficulties that are certain to meet them as they go out into life."

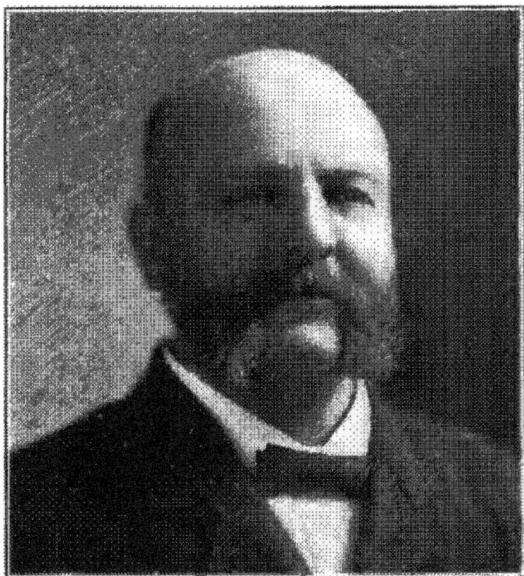

ANTHONY COMSTOCK.

Secretary of the New York Society for the Suppression of
Vice; author of " Frauds Exposed," " Traps for
the Young," etc.

"I have read the book ' What a Young Boy Ought
to Know ' with a great deal of interest, first, because
I am deeply impressed with the necessity for instructing the boys of the day; secondly, because what you
have presented is presented in such a way as to lift the
mind and thoughts upon a high and lofty plane upon
delicate subjects. I am satisfied that every parent who
has a boy would be benefited if he would carefully read
this book himself and then communicate the facts to
his boy, either by putting the book into the boy's hand
or using your methods as a medium for instructing the
boy about things which he ought to know. There is
a great demand for this book, and I hope it may be
blessed to the elevation of the thoughts and hearts of
the boys of this nation, and to the bringing in of a
better and higher social condition."

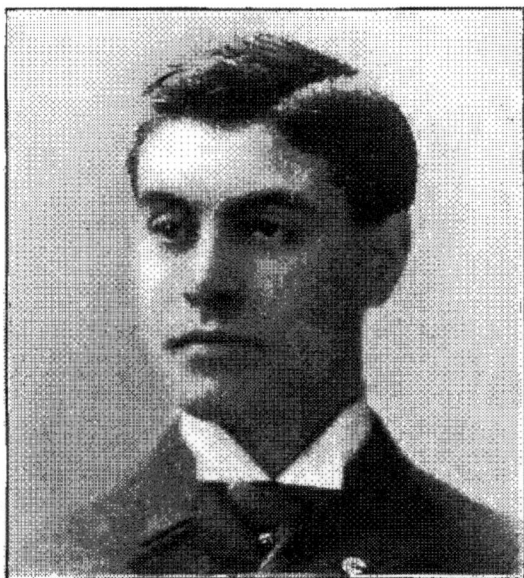

JOHN WILLIS BAER.

General Secretary of the United Society of Christian
Endeavor.

"If there is anything that I can say that will
stimulate the reading of Dr. Stall's book entitled
'What a Young Boy Ought to Know,' I am anxious
to say that word. I wish every parent might give
the book careful reading. I feel confident that it can
do great good, and I mean that my boys shall have
the contents placed before them. I am planning now
to read the book aloud to them."

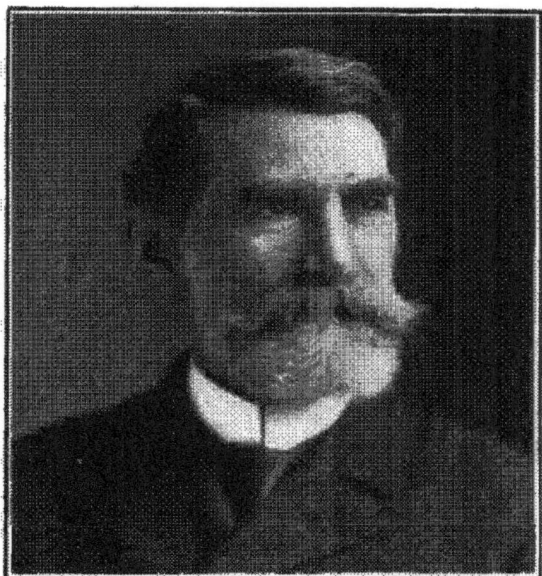

JOSIAH STRONG, D.D.

General Secretary of the Evangelical Alliance for the United States; author of "Our Country," "New Era," etc.

"Your treatment of a most delicate subject is eminently wise. Permit me to say that your method is precisely that which I employed a few years ago with my own boy. A foolish and culpable silence on the part of most parents leaves their children to learn, too often from vicious companions, sacred truth in an unhallowed way. Your book is most reverent and will inspire reverence. I hope many parents will have the wisdom to make use of it."

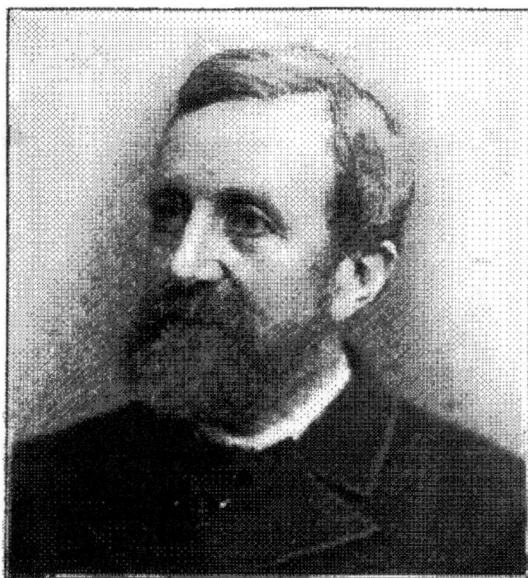

AARON M. POWELL.

Editor of *The Philanthropist;* President of the American
Purity Alliance.

" I have just finished reading the admirable book ' What a
Young Boy Ought to Know.' I regard it as a most valuable
addition to Purity literature, especially for boys and young
men. The reverential spirit with which it deals with the profoundly important subject of the sexual life cannot but prove
most helpful to the young who may be so fortunate as to come
under its educational influence. In view of the widespread
neglect of parents and teachers to give instruction along this
line to boys, many feeling incompetent to do it, and others
inclined to avoid the subject altogether, it will, properly
circulated, fill a large place of usefulness. Of its great need,
we are having continually only too many impressive and
painful object lessons in the blighted lives of many otherwise promising young men and in the ruined homes of
many who are older."

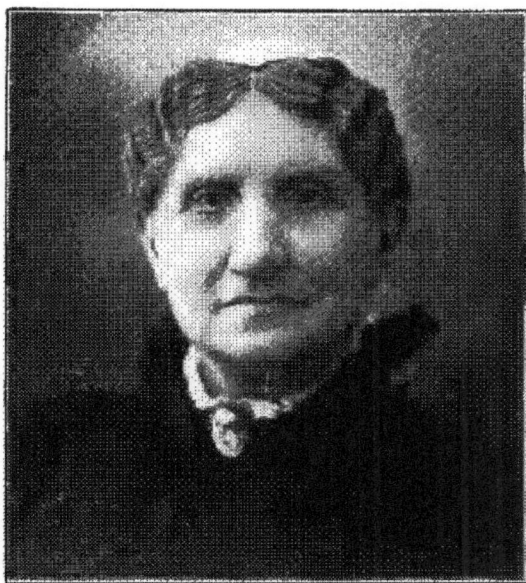

MRS. MARY A. LIVERMORE, LL.D.

Lecturer; author of " My Story of the War," " Woman of the Century," " The Story of My Life," etc.

" I have carefully read Dr. Stall's little book, ' What a Young Boy Ought to Know,' and am glad to commend it. He has treated the most delicate subjects so wisely that the most fastidious cannot object. The short chapters, full of physiological truths, which all children ought to know, at a proper age, will be read by boys without awakening a prurient thought ; and the warning against harmful habits and thoughts must prove a safeguard.''

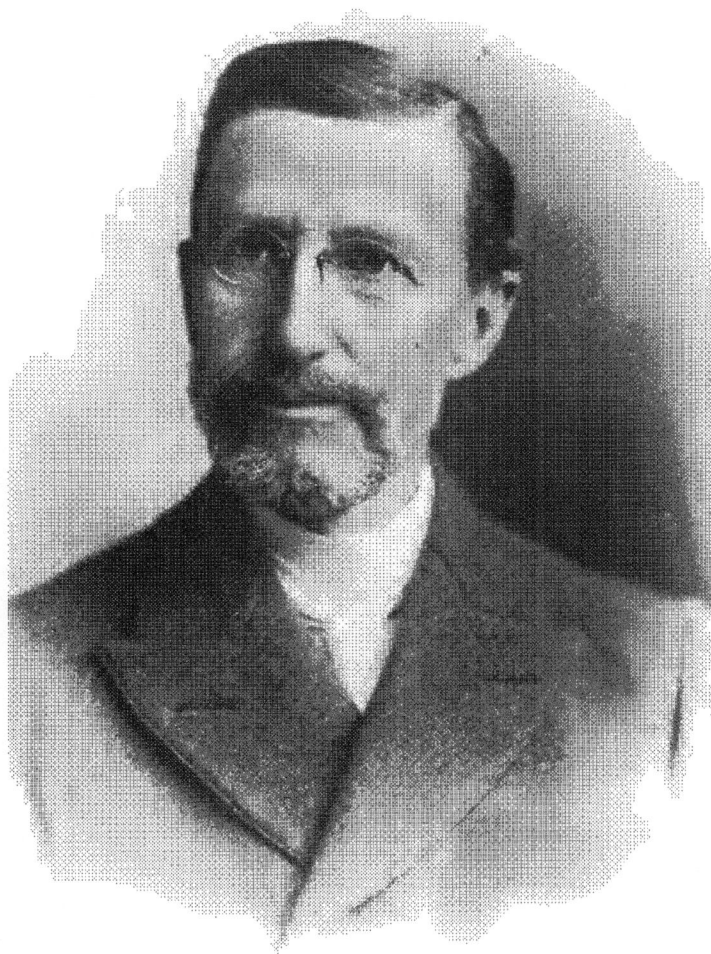

SYLVANUS STALL, D.D.

PRICE $1.00 NET
4s. NET

PURITY AND TRUTH

Self and Sex Series

WHAT A YOUNG BOY OUGHT TO KNOW

BY

SYLVANUS STALL, D. D.

Author of "What a Young Man Ought to Know," "What a
Young Husband Ought to Know," "What a Man of 45
Ought to Know," "Methods of Church Work," "Five-
Minute Object Sermons to Children," "Talks to
the King's Children," "Bible Selections for
Daily Devotion," etc., Associate Editor
of the "Lutheran Observer."

"IGNORANCE IS VICE."—*Socrates.*

PHILADELPHIA, PA.: 2237 LAND TITLE BUILDING

THE VIR PUBLISHING COMPANY

LONDON : 7, IMPERIAL ARCADE, LUDGATE CIRCUS, E. C.

TORONTO : WM. BRIGGS, 33 RICHMOND STREET, WEST

COPYRIGHT, 1897, BY SYLVANUS STALL

———

Entered at Stationers' Hall, London, England

Protected by International copyright in Great Britain and all
her colonies, and, under the provisions of the Berne Conven-
tion, in Belgium, France, Germany, Italy, Spain, Switzer-
land, Tunis, Hayti, Luxembourg, Monaco, Montenegro,
and Norway ———

[PRINTED IN THE UNITED STATES]

Dedicated

TO

THE THOUSANDS OF BOYS WHOSE HONEST INQUIRIES
CONCERNING THE ORIGIN OF LIFE AND BEING
DESERVE SUCH A TRUTHFUL, INTELLIGENT, AND
SATISFACTORY ANSWER AS WILL SAVE
THEM FROM IGNORANCE, ENABLE
THEM TO AVOID VICE, AND
DELIVER THEM FROM
SOLITARY AND SO-
CIAL SINS.

CONTENTS.

PART I.

GOD'S PURPOSE IN ENDOWING PLANTS, ANI-
MALS, AND MAN WITH REPRODUCTIVE
ORGANS.

CYLINDER I.

CYLINDER II.

3

CYLINDER V.

CYLINDER VI.

CYLINDER VII.

PART II.

THE MANNER IN WHICH THE REPRODUCTIVE ORGANS ARE INJURED IN BOYS BY ABUSE.

CYLINDER VIII.

Man is an Animal.—Has Intelligence, a
Moral Sense, and a Conscience.—How
the Intellect, Moral Sense, and Con-

PART III.

WHAT ARE THE CONSEQUENCES IN BOYS OF THE ABUSE OF THE REPRODUCTIVE ORGANS.

CYLINDER XI.

CYLINDER XII.

CYLINDER XIII.

PART IV.

HOW BOYS MAY PRESERVE THEIR ENTIRE BODIES IN PURITY AND STRENGTH.

CYLINDER XIV.

CYLINDER XV.

CYLINDER XVI.

CYLINDER XVII.

PART V.

PART VI.

PART VII.

THE AGE OF PUBERTY AND ITS ATTENDANT CHANGES.

CYLINDER XX.

CYLINDER XXI.

PREFACE.

WHEN himself a boy, the writer felt
the need of just such a book as this.
In later years, when a student in college,
and again afterward, when an active
pastor, he saw the need of a clean, pure,
but full-orbed and truthful book ad-
dressed to young men. Recognizing
this need, the writer resolved, more than
twenty years ago, that at some time in
the future, if God would fit him for the
difficult task, he would consecrate every
acquisition and talent to the faithful ac-
complishment of this delicate undertak-
ing. It was in the fulfillment of this purpose, which neither time nor manifold
divergent duties have ever obliterated or
even obscured that, just as the writer of
this little book was completing the manu-
script for a book to young men, the occasion arose for him to prepare and present

to young boys the thought which is embodied in this volume.

That there is need for such a book
as this no one who remembers his own
childhood, or who has carefully observed
the childhood of to-day, can have a rea-
sonable doubt. How successfully the
author has accomplished his delicate and
difficult task he must leave others to
judge. Wherein he has failed he hopes
that others may find that such failure is
in no measure due to the lack of a pure
and holy purpose.

Parents and literary critics will remember that this book is to young boys.
The language is designedly simple, and
in order that this important subject
might be more permanently impressed
upon the mind, we have not only avoided
such modes of expression as might conceal instead of reveal our meaning, but
have purposely sought, even at the risk
of repetition, to recall at certain intervals
such cardinal facts as seemed to us necessary to be kept before the mind for a
longer period.

This book is designed to be placed in
the hands of children who are, per-

chance, old enough to read for themselves, or, as in other cases, to be read
by the father or mother to the child.
Where a parent fears that his child might
ask promiscuous and embarrassing questions, it is well to say that such is not
likely to be the case, and if such ques-
tioning should arise, it will only be necessary to say to the child that if he will
be patient until the book is finished he
will doubtless have an answer to every
proper question upon this subject.

While this book is written primarily
to small boys, we believe it will be found
equally interesting to both men and
women, young and old.

We cannot but feel that the division of
our subject into separate treatises, suited
respectively in style and subject-matter
to boys and men in different periods and
conditions of life, will be found one of
the best features which has ever been
introduced into literature of this kind.
The mistake of placing in the hands of
a child a book containing information
which is designed only for grown persons is too obvious to need any discus-
sion. In this, as in an educational series,

the later books presuppose, and are in a large measure dependent upon the acquaintance of the reader with those which have gone before, but an intelligent understanding of none of the books is dependent upon any other book later in the series.

In so far as this little book shall meet the real needs of boys, merit the hearty approval of parents, and secure the rich blessing of heaven, the author will have attained the purpose which has been his inspiration.

SYLVANUS STALL.

PHILADELPHIA, PA.

INTRODUCTORY.

———

FOR a few moments each evening for more than a month Harry had been an attentive listener to a chapter from "Talks to the King's Children." One afternoon when he returned home from school he found Mamma's place in the nursery occupied by a strange, elderly lady and a little baby, which he was told was his baby sister. Being an intelligent, thoughtful boy, it was not unnatural that, with his mingled feelings of pleasure and perplexity, he should steal into his mother's room and, when they were alone, ask " Where did Baby come from? "

The parents have turned to the author of Harry's books for an answer to Harry's question, and here it is.

My Dear Friend Harry: I have received your Mamma's note, asking me to occupy her vacant place in the nursery for a few evenings, and in short Talks like the "five minute object sermons" to which you have been listening, tell you how God has created all who have lived upon the earth.

Distance and other circumstances render it impossible for me to come in person, and your Papa has consented that the phonograph shall be brought down from his study and placed in the nursery, so that each evening you may listen to a Talk, spoken into the phonograph which I have in my own study. So here is the first cylinder. I shall endeavor to speak distinctly, so that you may have no trouble in understanding, and will try to use plain, short words, so that a boy of your years may know my whole meaning, and have a truthful and satisfactory answer to your question.

When your Mamma's note came I was engaged in writing a book to young men on somewhat similar subjects, and your question is, therefore, in sympathy with my present thinking.

I send the first cylinder with this note of explanation. May God bless you and make you a pure and good man!

Your Sincere Friend,

SYLVANUS STALL.

PHILADELPHIA, PA.,
January 25, 1897.

PART L

God's Purpose in Endowing Plants, Animals, and
Man with Reproductive Organs.

WHAT A YOUNG BOY
OUGHT TO KNOW.

CYLINDER I.

The Question of the Origin of Life, Natural and Proper.—To Go Back to the Beginning. —The Account of Creation in Genesis.— Difference Between Making and Creating. —God Created Everything out of Nothing.— From Some Objects God Withheld the Power to Produce Others.—Upon Others He Bestowed Reproductive Power.—This Power Closely Resembles Creative Power.

MY DEAR FRIEND HARRY: The question you have asked is one that every man and woman, every intelligent boy and girl, and even many very young children have asked of themselves or others—whence and how they came to be in the world? The question is both natural and proper, and every intelligent person has a right to expect an answer that shall be truthful and, at the same time, told in such language that the meaning can be easily understood.

I am sure the boy is fortunate who has had intelligent parents or kind friends to give an honest and satisfactory answer to his question, and whose mind has been saved from the evil of those false and vile thoughts that are so general and common among ignorant men and boys.

If you were to ask where the locomotive and the steamship, or the telegraph and the telephone come from, it would seem to us wisest, in order that you might have the largest understanding of the subject and the fullest and most satisfactory answer, that we should go back to the beginning of these things, and consider what was done by George Stephenson and Robert Fulton, by Benjamin Franklin and Robert Morse, by Graham Bell and Thomas Edison toward developing and perfecting these useful inventions. In this way we are sure the most intelligent and complete understanding of the entire subject could be secured.

In order that we may, in like manner,

have the best understanding of the answer to the question, " Where did we come from? " let us, in the same way, go back and ask where did Adam, the first man, and Eve, the first woman, come from? Of course you already know that God created Adam and Eve. You have read the beautiful and wonderful account given on the first page of the Bible; but there are many things in this wonderful account in the book of Genesis which you have doubtless overlooked. Let us for a few moments study this account together.

If we start with the first verse we are told that, " In the beginning God created the heavens and the earth." Now there is a great difference between creating and making anything. When a carpenter builds, or makes a house or a barn, he simply brings together boards, bricks, shingles, laths, nails, and other things, and with these he erects the building; but when it is all completed he has not created anything. He has simply taken those things which previously existed, and so changed their form and combined them as to make what we call a building. In other words, he has built a building. He has created nothing, but he has made something.

With God it was not so. In the beginning, when God created everything, there were no rocks, no ground, no materials of any kind with which He could build or make the world, or anything else. But God's power and wisdom were without limit, and instead of using materials, or even needing materials to accomplish His purpose, He simply commanded, and it was done. There was endless and dense darkness, and God simply said "Let there be light; and there was light." On the second day God created the firmament, or the blue expanse above us, and so, for six days, God went on creating all that exists upon the earth, all that swims in the seas, that flies in the air, and that shines in the sky.

To some of the works of His creation God gave the power to beget or produce others like themselves. Such objects learned men call organic objects. From some others, which learned men call inorganic objects, such as the sun, moon, stars, rocks, mountains, oceans, and the like, God withheld that power to produce others. These latter are to abide until God shall destroy them, and hence it was not necessary that they should have given to them power to produce others like themselves. If other worlds should be needed, God prefers to create them Himself. But the other objects, which learned men call organic objects, the things which have life, such as plants, trees, fishes, birds, animals, and men, these do not abide or remain continually, but live only for a time and then die and pass away.

Now when this is the case, God could from time to time create others to take their places, and thus cause that life should continue upon the earth. But God saw a wiser and better way, and in infinite wisdom and love He gave to all the objects and creatures which He created, and which He endowed with life, the power to beget and reproduce others like themselves. It was not power to create as God had Himself so wonderfully and mysteriously done; but it was a power which in some respects resembles it very closely, and which in its deepest mystery the wisest men have never yet been able fully to understand or explain. It was a power to impart life; to beget and to produce others like themselves.

This, Harry, is the wonderful subject which you and I have set ourselves reverently to study. In order that we may have an intelligent and satisfactory answer to the question, " Where did we and each person who lives upon the earth come from? " it will be necessary to study the Bible account of creation a little more in detail, and this we will do to-morrow night.

CYLINDER II.

The Creation of Plants, Animals, and Man, Each after His Kind.—How God Created Adam and Eve.—The Bible Account.—Reproductive Power Ordained of God.—God Would Not Make a Law that Had Impurity in It.—If We Do Not Blush at the Manner in Which God Created Adam and Eve, Neither Should We at the Manner in Which He Created Cain and Abel.—Thinking God's Pure Thoughts after Him.—Reproductive Resembles Creative Power.

MY DEAR FRIEND HARRY: I want to talk to you to-night about how in the beginning God created Adam and Eve, and ordained that the life of plants, animals, and man should be perpetuated Now if we turn again to the first chapter of Genesis, we find that on the third day God created the grass and herbs, " Each yielding seed, and the fruit tree yielding fruit after his kind, whose seed is in itself." On the fifth day He created the fishes and birds, " and God blessed them saying, Be fruitful, and multiply." And on the sixth day He created " Cattle and creeping things, and beasts of the earth, after his kind." And last of all, in the work of creation, God also created man.

Now if we take the different verses from the first and second chapters of Genesis, and bring them together in a continuous account, the history of man's creation in God's own words will read: " God said, Let us make man in our image, after our likeness, and let them have dominion over the fish of the sea, and over the fowl of the air, and over the cattle, and over all the earth, and over every creeping thing that creepeth upon the earth. And the LORD God formed man *of* the dust of the ground, and breathed into his nostrils the breath of life; and man became a living soul. And the LORD God planted a garden eastward in Eden; and there He put the man whom He had formed. And the LORD God said, *It is* not good that the man should be alone; I will make him a help meet for him. And the LORD God caused a deep sleep to fall upon Adam, and he slept; and He took one of his ribs, and closed up the flesh instead thereof. And the rib, which the LORD God had taken from man, made He a woman, and brought her unto the man. And Adam said, This *is* now bone of my bones, and flesh of my flesh: she shall be called Woman, because she was taken out of man. Therefore shall a man leave his father and his mother, and shall cleave unto his wife: and they shall be one flesh. So God created man in His *own* image, in the image of God created He him; male and female created He them. And God blessed them, and God said unto them, Be fruitful, and multiply, and replenish the earth, and subdue it: and have dominion over the fish of the sea, and over the fowl of the air, and over every living thing that moveth upon the earth."

I am sure, my dear boy, that you will agree with me that this is a very beautiful account, and in it we have a revelation of God's mind and method of raising up or producing others to take the places of all the plants, trees, fishes, birds, animals, and men which God had created upon the earth, but which would all, in a few years, die and pass away.

This law or method by which parent plants and animals beget, or raise up, infant plants and animals, like themselves, to occupy their places, and thus continue life upon the earth after they are dead and gone, we are here clearly taught was instituted or ordained by God himself, and we know that God would not make a law that had impurity in it.

Now we do not blush or regard it impure to study the wonderful wisdom and power which God displayed in the creation of Adam and Eve. Neither should we, when we think properly of the no less wonderful and mysterious manner in which God created Cain and Abel, their children, and in which He still is from day to day and year to year, raising up a new generation to take the places of their parents, when they shall have died and passed away. If we remember that no impure thought ever entered into the mind of our dear heavenly Father, when He was thinking of these things, and when engaged in the work of creation, we will clearly understand that all wrong thinking or acting upon this subject, which should be as pure and sacred to our minds as any other sacred subject, comes from Satan, and not from God. If we truly realize this we shall then be in the proper frame of mind to ask God that we may, upon this subject, think His thoughts after Him, in the same pure way that He thought them at the time of the creation, and before the creation, and since the creation. If we get our thoughts from God, they will be pure, and if we get them from Satan they will be impure. In itself the subject is pure, and we should bring to its consideration a reverent and devout mind.

You will have noticed in this account that God gave to plants, trees, and every living creature, the power to produce others, each of their own kind. Had they not been thus limited or restricted, peaches might have grown upon apple trees, and chestnuts might have grown upon currant bushes. Neither were they permitted to exercise creative power as God had done, else trees might have created fishes or birds, and birds might have created trees or animals, according to pleasure. But each was given power to produce and perpetuate his own kind by bearing " Seed after his kind." On this account apple seeds, when properly planted, always produce apple trees, and peach seeds always produce peach trees, and so on through all the forms of life and being. So God endowed plants and animals, and every living creature, not with creative power, but with another power which in some respects, as we have said, resembles it very closely, and which, because each produces seed after its own kind, and from these seeds grow up or are produced baby plants which are like the parent plants, we call this power, not creative power, but reproductive power.

The manner in which this power is seen in plants, I shall try to tell you on the next cylinder.

CYLINDER III.

Father, Mother, and Baby Plants.—'' Male and Female Created He Them.''—The Father and Mother Natures in the Same Stalk.—Seen only at Maturity of Stalk in the Production of the Seed.—Seen in the Cornfield.—The Ears with the Silk the Female, and the Tassels with the Pollen the Male Manifestation.— The Father and Mother Natures Sometimes Separated.—The Pollen Carried by the Wind and Insects.—Were God to Destroy the Reproductive Power of Plants and Trees, all Vegatable Life Would Disappear and Animals and Men Would Die of Starvation.

My Dear Friend Harry: At the close of my little Talk to you in the phonograph last evening, I spoke of the young plant that grows up from the seed which is planted in the ground, and I called it, the " baby plant." A plant is just as truly a child of its parents as the little birds in the nest are the children of the parent birds which built the nest, hatched out the baby birds, and afterward

37

watched over and fed them so tenderly. In the case of the birds you may have noticed that there were two parent birds, the father bird and the mother bird. But in the account of the creation in the book of Genesis, you may have failed to notice the full meaning in the place where it tells of the different living things which God created, and it says, " Male and female created He them." This fact you doubtless have noticed with animals, and possibly with birds, but you may not have thought that God designed that each baby plant should also have both a father and a mother, and that concerning plants it is also true, "male and female created He them." Such, however, is the real fact.

In some plants, the father and the mother natures dwell together in the same parent stalk, but are seen in their separate father and mother natures only when the period of full growth and maturity has come in the life of the plant, and seed is to be produced, so that, later on, when the parent plant shall wither and die, other young plants may spring up from the seed, and thus, although the parent plant has died and passed away, yet by means of the seed, the life of that kind of plant is preserved and continued upon the earth.

The manner in which these father and mother natures are united, and yet show themselves separately in the work of forming the seed from which the baby plant is afterward to grow, is perhaps most easily seen in a field where corn, or what English boys call Indian corn is growing. After the stalk is grown to its full height, and the ears have begun to form, and spread out that fine silk which you have no doubt noticed at the upper ends of the ears, at the same time there also appeared upon the top of the stalk a great number of blossoms, which boys generally call tassels. Now these ears, with their husks, out of which hang the silk, are the mother, or the female manifestations of the plant, and the tassels with their blossoms covered with pollen, or flower dust, are the father or male manifestations of the plant. When a gentle breeze shakes the corn stalk, and the pollen, or fine flower dust falls from the tassels upon the silk, it is carried by

separate threads of silk to each separate
kernel, and in this way each grain
growing upon the entire stalk has imparted to it that principle of life, without
which it could never become a grain of
corn.

In all plants, the father and mother
natures are manifested in the flower, and
are seen in the blossoms upon the trees
and the roses upon the bushes. In some
instances the two natures, as in the case
of corn, are united in the same tree or
bush; while in others, the father and
mother natures live in separate trees or
in separate bushes. When they are
found together in the same flower, the
pollen, or flower dust from the male
anthers is easily conveyed to the female
stigma, and thus passes down the style,
or stem, to the pod, which is hidden
away beneath the beautiful leaves of the
flower, where the seeds, after being
made by the pollen to have the principle
of life, are to grow to maturity. In some
cases, the male and female natures are
found in separate blossoms or flowers,
sometimes on the same branch, and at
other times upon separate branches of

the same plant. In other instances, they grow only upon separate trees, and these papa and mamma trees with their blossoms may be growing, not close together, but widely apart from each other, separated sometimes as far as you can throw a stone, and at other times with broad fields lying between them, or even several miles apart. Where they are separated by some distance, the pollen, or flower dust of the male, or father blossom, is carried to the blossoms of the female, or mother plant by the wind and by bees and other insects which have no thought of doing the blossoms this kind service, but are only anxious and intent on gathering honey to be stored away for their winter food.

By what I have said you will understand something of the wisdom which God displayed, when in the beginning He created plants and trees, each "Yielding seed after his kind," and also how God is to-day reproducing, perpetuating, and distributing the life of every herb, every blade of grass, of every flower and of every tree, to take the places of those herbs, plants, and trees, which are soon to wither, die, and pass away. If God were to withhold from all forms of plants and trees the power to exercise this wonderful reproductive power with which He has endowed them, only a few years at most would pass away, until every green thing would have died and perished from the earth, and there would be no flowers or fruit, no grain or food of any kind, and famine and death would sweep every bird and beast, and even man himself, from the face of the entire earth.

Thus, Harry, you will see that by thinking of these things in the same pure way which God shows us in the Bible, we are coming, step by step, to the full and satisfactory answer to the question which you asked of your dear Mamma when you came home the other evening and found your innocent, sweet baby sister lying in the cradle.

To-morrow night, I will tell you how God provided that every baby fish, and bird, and baby animal, should also have a papa and mamma.

CYLINDER IV.

MY DEAR FRIEND HARRY: On the
former cylinders I tried to tell you, as
you will remember, how that when God
created the sun, moon, stars, rocks,
mountains, seas, and all such things as
learned men call inorganic objects He did
not give them power to produce others
like themselves, but reserved to himself
the power either to destroy, or to create
others, as He might deem best. I told
you also how that among herbs, trees,

43

and all objects which have life, and which learned men call organic objects, God gave the power to produce others like themselves, but these new products were to begin life as infants. In the instance of all plants, vegetables, and grain, this process goes on repeating itself. Starting with the plant, of each kind, which God created, there was next the blossom or flower, then the fruit or seed, and these seeds in turn producing other similar infant plants, and these when grown, in their turn also blossomed and produced seeds, and so on from the first, the process repeating itself down to the present; each plant and tree preparing the way for the continuation of its own life in the plant or tree which was to come after it, and so on and on, through all the years to the end of time.

By recalling these things we shall be prepared, to-night, on this cylinder, to go one step further. Now the forms of organic life, for simplicity and convenience, are divided into two classes. One class, because they have nerves and some one or more of the five senses of hearing, seeing, smelling, tasting, and feeling are called sentient or feeling beings. The other class, composed of such objects as plants and trees, which we have already considered, and which have no nerves, and do not have any of the five senses, are called non-sentient or not-feeling beings.

When we come to birds, fishes, and all kinds of animals, instead of the papa and mamma natures uniting in the production of seeds, as is the case in plants, they unite in producing an egg. Some eggs, like those of birds, are covered with a shell, but that is not the case with all eggs. Instead of the papa nature, producing pollen, as in plants, in creat-·ures that have nerves, a watery fluid takes the place of the pollen, and this is imparted to that portion of the egg which the mamma parent produces in various ways, as we shall see presently.

First let us take the oyster, which can neither hear, see, smell, nor possibly taste, and because it has only the single sense of feeling is regarded as one of the lowest in the scale of development of all the sentient beings; and we will find that, like most of the plants, both the father and mother natures dwell together in the person of a single oyster, and while the egg is being formed in the body of the parent oyster, the father and mother each contribute their part, so as to produce what is called a fertile egg, or one that will produce a baby oyster. When these eggs are fully formed, which occurs in the spring of the year, they are expelled from the body of the parent oyster, and float about in the water until they rest against a rock, the shell of a large oyster, or some other hard substance, to which they at once lay hold, and immediately the shell, which constitutes both the oyster's house and clothing, begins to grow and forms about its little body.

With fish, it is different. When God created the fishes, He gave the mamma nature a separate body of its own, and he also gave the papa nature a separate body of its own. So the baby fish, like baby boys and girls, has two parents; one the mamma fish, and the other the papa fish.

I suppose that in the spring of the year, when Mamma has ordered a large shad sent home, and Bridget was cleaning it, you may have noticed that its body was filled with thousands of eggs. These are often cooked with the fish, and are called " roes." Now during most of the year, these shad live in deep sea-water, and in the spring when their bodies are thus full of the eggs which have formed during the year, all the shad leave their regular home, and swim into the bays, or sometimes hundreds of miles up the river, until they find some quiet, safe, and suitable place where the mamma fishes may lay their eggs, or " spawn," as it is called. It is while on this journey up the rivers in the spring of the year, that many of the shad are caught by fishermen in great nets. On this journey, the mamma fishes are accompanied by the papa fishes, and when the suitable place which they are seeking is found, the mamma fishes expel from their bodies those thousands of eggs, which are at the same time accompanied by and float in a slimy substance that very much resembles the white portion of a raw hen's egg. After the mamma fish has thus laid her eggs, the papa fish swims gently over the eggs, at the same time expelling from his body a slimy substance which also resembles the white portion of a raw hen's egg.   In this way the eggs are fertilized, the same as the grains of corn are fertilized by having the pollen, or flower dust, fall upon the silk at the end of the ear, and which is carried by the silk threads down under the husk to each separate grain of corn on the stalk.

After the eggs of the fishes have been thus deposited in the water where the conditions are favorable, the parents go away, and never see, or at least never know their baby fishes, which are hatched in a few days by the motion of the water and the warmth of the sun. Both baby fishes and baby oysters are little orphans from the very beginning.

So you see where the baby fishes come from, and to-morrow evening, I will tell you about baby birds and baby animals.

CYLINDER V.

How Seeds Are Made to Grow.—How Eggs
Are Hatched.—The Habits of Parent Birds
While Hatching.—The Beautiful Lessons
They Teach.—The Dangers to which Little
Birds Are Exposed.—Their Return from
Sunny Climes to Build Nests of Their Own.
—Animals Next in the Order of Creation.—
Reasons Why Animals Do Not Lay Eggs.—
The Egg Retained in the Body of the Mother
Animal.—Her Body Marvelously Furnished.
—After Sufficient Growth the Young Animal
is Born.—After Birth, Still Nourished from
the Mother's Body.—Weaned when the
Teeth Grow.—Lowest Animals Reach
Bodily Maturity Soonest.—Man Highest in
the Scale of Being.—Longest of All in
Reaching Maturity.—Value of Childhood
Years.

MY DEAR FRIEND HARRY: I prom-
ised to tell you to-night about baby birds
and baby animals. In the spring of the
year you have gone with Mamma into
the garden and seen her plant the seeds
of flowers and vegetables. After she
dropped these seeds, she covered them
carefully so that the moisture of the

earth and the warmth of the sun might waken the life which was dormant or sleeping in the seeds, and in which the infant plants were all enfolded ready to awake and grow up, first into baby plants, and then into big plants.

When you have seen the little eggs in the nest which the birds built in the tree near your window, did it occur to you that these were the seeds out of which should come new birds. Such, in fact, however, the eggs really are. But instead of being placed in the earth like the seeds of plants, the parent birds build a nest where they can sit on the eggs, impart to them the warmth of their own bodies, and thus quicken or awaken the life which is in the eggs, so that the bodies of the little birds might form and grow as God has ordained. In this way, after two or three weeks, when the birds are grown large enough, the shell breaks open, and the tiny little birds are then born, or hatched, as we say.

If you have carefully watched the two parent birds during the weeks while the little birds were being hatched, you will have noticed that the mamma bird pre-

fers to sit most of the time on the eggs
and keep them warm, but all the while
the papa bird has stayed close by, coming often to sit on a branch near the
nest, and chirp and sing, and thus cheer
and keep the mamma bird company,
then he would fly away, and after a little
time return, carrying in his beak a
worm, or some choice bit of food which
he had found, and flying up to the nest,
feed it lovingly to the mamma bird. At
times, when the mamma bird was tired,
they would both fly away together, and
after a few moments, the papa bird
would hurry back to take the mamma
bird's place, and keep the eggs warm
and guard them from harm, while the
mamma bird would take such rest and
recreation as she needed or wished.

The home life of two such parent birds
is very devoted and sweet, and no man
or boy can watch it without learning
from the birds lessons of love and
fidelity.

While the little birds are growing, the
parent birds unite in hunting food, and
after the baby birds have attained some
size, and their feathers are grown, then

the parent birds have an anxious time, lest the ambitious little birds too soon attempt to fly, only to fall on the ground and be caught by the cat, or die after a period of mishaps and misfortunes. If the little birds are only patient, they will, in due time, fly safely from tree to tree, and after spending the summer in the neighborhood of their babyhood home, will then fly away to spend the winter in a warm clime, and if not shot by some heartless and cruel man or boy who is gunning, they will return the next spring fully grown and matured, and with their own mates will also take their places in the reproductive world, and as God has ordained in this succession of life, build nests for themselves and their mates in the neighboring trees, and raise up for themselves a brood of baby birds.

Now next in the order and scale of creation come the animals. Animals do not lay eggs like birds, and for good reasons. You remember how it is with the fishes. Many produce thousands of eggs in a single season. Some codfish have been known to contain as many as sixteen or twenty millions of eggs at one time. Many of these eggs, after having been laid, because of unfavorable conditions, may never hatch, and of such as are hatched, vast multitudes of them are devoured by the larger fish, for fish are cannibals, and eat their own kind. The eggs of birds are also exposed to various forms of danger and destruction, as in the case of ducks, geese, and chickens, whose eggs are one of the forms of food designed to sustain human life.

To prevent such loss, and to accomplish other beneficent ends, when we come to the higher forms of life, we find that instead of laying the eggs in a nest, and then sitting upon them until the young are hatched, with animals, the egg, after being fertilized by the sexual contact of the male, is retained in the body of the mother. Here, in a portion of her body, which God has marvelously fashioned and furnished for that purpose, changes similar to those which occur in the egg while the mother bird is sitting upon it take place in the development and growth of the egg while it yet remains in the body of the mother animal. After a time, varying from a few months to an entire year, as when the little chick, after having attained sufficient development, breaks the shell and comes forth to begin its own independent life, so the egg or germ which has been retained in the body of the mother animal, when it is developed and grown sufficiently to live its own separate and independent life, comes forth from its mother's body, and is born, as we say. Until the time that it is born, it is nourished within the body of the mother, but after it is born, God still supplies the nourishment from the body of the mother, but no longer upon the inner side of the mother's body, but upon the outside of her body, where the young obtain it in the form of milk.

In this way, the young animal is usually fed for a few weeks, after which it is furnished with teeth, and is then weaned, as we say. After it is weaned, it enters upon a further stage of growth, requiring, as it is higher or lower in the scale of being, months or even years to attain its full growth and maturity. The lower in the scale of being, the briefer the period of babyhood and childhood, and the higher in the scale of being, the longer that period, and the more time it takes to complete the growth, and arrive at a state of full bodily maturity.

Now man is the highest in the scale of being, and consequently his period of childhood and growth is longest of all the creatures that God has created. But we must remember that God has made man ruler over all else that He has created, and it is therefore necessary that he should have many years of growth in order that he might be taught, and gain knowledge, experience, and wisdom, so that, when he should reach his full maturity, he may be endowed with fullest powers, as God has ordained, so that he might be worthy of the high place which God has assigned him as ruler over all else that He has created, and be worthy to stand in the scale of being next to God Himself, in whose likeness and image man was created.

My dear boy, like many others you may often have wished that you might sooner become a man. But God surely

knows best, and the years which still lie
between this and the time when, at
twenty-five years of age, you shall have
reached your full bodily maturity, is not
too long in order that you may be fully
prepared to bear life's burdens, and to
discharge all of man's serious responsibilities. Even though, in your own
home, you enjoy exceptional opportuni-
ties and advantages, yet like all boys you
will need to be both patient and indus-
trious, that these valuable years may not
be wasted, but properly improved.

CYLINDER VI.

Had God Created All as He Did Adam and Eve, Our Present Conditions and Relations Could Not Exist.—There Would Be No Homes, Parents, or Children.—No Childhood with Plays and Pleasures.—All Plans Were Open to God.—He Chose the Best Plan.—God Gave Man Power Similar to His Creative Power.—Purity of Parentage.—Why Parents Love Their Children.—The Twain Made One in Their Children.—The Human Egg, or Ovum.—The Male Life Germ.—How Life is Begotten.—Conversation of Mother and Child.—The Study of the Subject Begets Awe and Reverence.—The Wisest Cannot Fully Understand or Explain our Beginning and Growth.

MY DEAR FRIEND HARRY: Starting with the plants, night by night I have talked to you of fishes, birds, and animals, and to-night we are to consider how God has ordained that the life of man should be perpetuated upon the earth.

If God had created each individual

separately, full-sized men and women, without parents, and without a childhood, all the conditions of our lives would be different from what they now are. There would be no homes, for all the relations of life upon which the home now rests could not exist. There would be no relations such as husband and wife, father and mother, parent and child, brother and sister, aunts, uncles, cousins, and no grandpas or grandmas. Each individual would stand independently and unrelated to any and all others. The loves and affections which now give to life its sweetest charm and its noblest inspiration, would be entirely lacking. Instead of being as links in an unbroken succession of life, you and I and each individual would stand alone with no one to share our joys, to help us bear our burdens, to minister to our needs, to watch over us as our parents and friends now do in sickness, or to mourn our loss at death. There would be no sweet little babies, with dimpled cheeks and chubby chins, no childhood, with its plays and pleasures, no school days, and no gradual unfolding of the mind and needed preparation for life's purpose and work.

All plans for creating the first people who should live upon the earth, and those who should come afterward to take their places, were open to God. He was not limited by any one or even many ways of doing this, for all wisdom and all power belong to Him. But God saw that for Him to go on creating men would not be the best plan. God wanted to bring man very close to Himself and so God gave man the power to transmit life; the power to receive life from parents, and in later years to hand it down to their own children. In order that this might be accomplished, when God created Adam and Eve, "male and female created He them," and endowed them with this marvelous power, and intrusted this power to them as a sacred gift.

So you see, my dear friend Harry, that the question which relates to sex, concerning which thoughtless boys and wicked men think and speak so vulgarly and lewdly is, after all, to be thought and spoken of only with reverence and purity. God made men and women to differ. He gave to woman her graceful figure, and a sense of dependence; and He gave to man his broader shoulders and greater strength, in order that man might guard, defend, and protect woman, not only from outward physical danger, but from every impurity of thought, word, and deed. No boy or man can think irreverently of the subjects which relate to sex without dishonoring God and wronging himself.

As you have seen the mutual interest of the parent birds in the care and well-being of the baby birds in the nests, so you daily experience the love and affection of your parents in many ways, and if you are the very thoughtful boy that I have taken you to be, you may possibly have asked yourself the question why Papa and Mamma love you so much as to have actual pleasure in doing such things as no others upon earth would be willing or even able to do for you in such a devoted and loving way. I will tell you why. It is because in you Mamma and Papa find a reproduction of themselves. You are part of them. You are not only part of Mamma, because in some senses God gave you first to her, and in that divine and mysterious way unfolded within her body that which was to constitute all the members of your body " When as yet there was none of them," but Papa likewise loves you because you are part of his body also. You have likely read in the Bible where it speaks of the husband and wife, and says, " And they twain," or two, " shall be one flesh," and so your Papa and Mamma are made one in you, and again in the little sister who so recently came to your home in the manner in which God ordained, and which He has instituted as the means of binding fathers, mothers, and children very closely to each other, and drawing all unitedly very close to Himself.

I have already told you that since the creation all forms of life begin with an egg. This is true also of human life. But the egg, or ovum, as it is called when formed in the body of a woman, is very small; so small indeed that it is not large enough to be seen unless placed under a magnifying glass. The same is true also of the spermatozoa or life germs, contained in the fluid called semen which forms in the body of a man, and by which, in the state of pure and holy marriage, God has ordained that the ovum, while yet in the body of the wife, shall be fertilized by the requisite and proper bodily contact of the husband, and that without such contact, the ovum or egg should never produce life.

In order that you may more fully understand the mystery of the beginning of life I am going to read to you from a booklet written by Dr. Mary Wood-Allen, who is a noble, pure-minded woman, and a devoted Christian mother, and who narrates the following conversation between a thoughtful little boy and a mother who wisely prefers to teach her child the truth rather than to leave him to the polluting influences of the school or the street.

" Mamma, how big was I when I was made? " asked a little boy.

" When you were made, my dear, you were but a tiny speck, not so big as the point of a needle. You could not

have been seen except with a micro-
scope."

"Why, Mamma, if I was as small as
that I should think I would have been
lost."

"So you would, dear child, if the kind
Heavenly Father had not taken especial
care of you. He knew how precious
little babies are, and so He has made
a little room in the mother's body, where
they can be kept from all harm until
they are big enough to live their own
separate lives."

"And did I live in such a little room
in you?"

"Yes, dear."

"But how did I eat and breathe?"

"I ate and breathed for you."

"Did you know I was there?"

"Yes. Sometimes your little hand or
foot would knock on the wall of the
room, and I would feel it and would say,
'My darling speaks to me and says,
"Mother, I am here"'; and then I
would say, 'Good-morning, little one,
mother loves you'; and then I would try
to think how you would look when I
should see you."

" How long was I there, Mamma? "

" Three-quarters of a year, and you grew and grew every day, and, because I wanted you to be happy, I tried to be happy all the time, and I was careful to eat good food so that you might be strong, and I tried to be gentle, kind, patient, persevering, in fact, everything that I wanted you to be, for I knew that everything I did would help to make you what you were to be."

" But Mamma, how did what you ate feed me? "

" My food was made into blood, and the blood was carried to you and nourished you."

" But how? "

" Did you ever see Mamma make a dumpling? "

" Yes. You took the dough and put the apple in and gathered the dough all up in one place and pinched it together."

" Yes, and you are much like a dumpling. Your skin is folded around you like the dough around the apple and is gathered together in one place on the front of the body. We call it the navel or umbilicus. Before you were born

the skin at this point was continued in
a long cord which was connected with
Mamma, and through it the blood was
carried to you. When the time came
for you to go out into the world to live
apart from me, the door of your little
room opened with much pain and suffering to me, and then you came into the
world, or were born, as we say. Then
the cord, or tube, that connected you to
me was cut, and, healing up, formed the
navel or the place where the skin of the
whole body is gathered together. When
you drew your first breath into your
lungs, you cried, and then I knew you
were alive and I laughed, and said, ' Is
it a boy or girl?' After you were washed
and dressed they brought you to me and
laid you on my arm and, for the first
time, I saw the face of the little baby I
had loved so long. And now you can
understand why you are so dear to me."

"Oh, Mamma, now I know why I
love you best of all the world," ex-
claimed the child, with warm embraces
and with loving tears in his eyes.

I am sure, dear Harry, that no one
can properly study the mystery of the

origin of life without having quickened in him a feeling of awe and reverence. In this whole matter God works in such marvelous mystery that not even the wisest man that ever lived can either fully understand or explain it.

On this cylinder and those which have preceded it, you now have what I have tried, as far as I have been able, to make a true, full, and satisfactory answer to the question which a couple of weeks ago you asked of your Mamma, and which, at your Mamma's request, I undertook to answer. There is one question which stands closely related to what we have been considering, and before bidding you good-by, I will to-morrow night call your attention to it.

CYLINDER VII.

Papa's Request to Continue the Talks.—Why
Children Look Like Their Parents.—Parents
Transmit Both Bodily and Mental Character-
istics.—Unhealthy Parents Cannot Have
Healthy Children.—What the Boy is, Deter-
mines What the Man Shall Be, and What
His Children Shall Be.—The Boy's Duty to
Those Who Are to Come after Him.—A
Good Inheritance No Occasion for Boasting.
—" Heredity Not Fatality."—Duty to Im-
prove What We Have.

My Dear Friend Harry: A letter
received from your Papa to-day has been
to me the source of much pleasure. He
also has listened to the cylinders which
I have sent you each evening, and with
kind expressions of appreciation and approval, has asked me to continue my
Talks along some related lines of
thought, which I trust may prove both
suggestive and of real value to you. I
have granted his request, and to-morrow
evening will begin a few Talks on some
abuses of the reproductive organs, and

how boys may preserve their entire bodies in purity and strength.

From what I told you in the phonograph last night, you will, I think, be able fully to understand why children so often look like their parents, act like them, think like them—are so much like them in many respects that we frequently hear the expression, " He is a chip of the old block."

God has not only ordained that every plant shall bear seed " after his kind," but shall also transmit to its successors its own minor characteristics. When you plant pop-corn, the seed will not grow to be some great tall variety of corn, neither when you set the eggs of bantams will they hatch leghorns or light brahmas. The corn and the little chicks will grow to be much like their parents. So it is with children. Their bodily beginning is in many ways a gift from their parents, in which the natures of papa and mamma are united, and on this account the child is the embodiment of both. Sometimes the child resembles one parent in looks and the other in character. Sometimes the color of the

child's eyes are like the eyes of the
father; in others like those of the mother;
while in other instances, the color of the
eyes of the child may be an expression
of the combined influence of both parents, or even of its grandparents. The
same is true of the color, quantity, and
quality of the hair, and of the other
physical manifestations which go so far
toward making up the looks of a person.

What is true of the looks is true also
of the health which parents transmit
to their children. Where fathers and
mothers do not have good health themselves they cannot transmit or give good
health to their children. If the parents
have weak, sickly, or diseased bodies the
children will be like them in this respect.
You will see, then, how important it is
that fathers and mothers should have
good health if they desire to have
healthy, cheerful, and happy children.
But if people desire to have good health
to transmit to their children they must
preserve their health while they are
young. What is done during boyhood
determines what shall be the condition
during manhood. What the boy is and

does will determine what the man shall be later on. And so, Harry, if you do not take care of your health, or if you do anything now to injure it, then, in later years, when you shall yourself become a father, your children will be sure to suffer the results of your negligence and imprudence.

The same is true of mental characteristics. In this also children receive their inheritance from their parents. In character, some children resemble one parent; in others there are some resemblances to both, while, in other instances, a child may inherit the result of the combined influences which have come down through a generation or two.

If these things are true, as they unquestionably are, then you see how influences which exerted themselves long years before you were born have all centered and wrought together to make you what you were when you were born. And so, in like manner, what you are now, while a boy, and what you shall grow to be in physical strength, in bodily health, in mind, and character, that your children shall largely become hereafter.

If you are gentle, kind, and truthful, it will be easier for them to be gentle, kind, and truthful. If you were to be disobedient, cruel, and deceitful, you would, by your conduct, make it difficult for them not to do the same things; but if you cheerfully obey your parents, honor and love them, and love and serve God, you will make it easier for your children to love and obey you, and to be faithful and upright Christian boys and girls.

You will see from what I have said to-night something of what the Bible means where it says that "No man liveth to himself, and no man dieth to himself." We stand related to the generations which have preceded us, and we owe a duty to the generations that shall come after us.

You have been blessed with good physical and intellectual powers, and this should be to you the occasion for great thankfulness, and not for boasting. Neither should those of us who have strong bodies think uncharitably and without sympathy of those who have received an inheritance of physical infirmities. We should also remember that

"Heredity is not fatality." Although we have received strong bodies, yet we may ruin them by abuse, and so, in like manner, by care and perseverance, those who have weaker bodies and less vigorous minds may acquire much, and even surpass those who received more by nature or inheritance. Our great care should be to improve all we have, and to see to it that those who come after us shall suffer nothing because of our sin or folly.

PART II.

The Manner in which the Reproductive Organs
are Injured in Boys by Abuse.

CYLINDER VIII.

Man is an Animal.—Has Intelligence, a Moral
Sense, and a Conscience.—How the Intellect,
Moral Sense, and Conscience are Dwarfed
and Blunted.— Comparative Anatomy.—
Points of Resemblance in Bodies of Man
and Four-footed Animals.—Between Man
and Birds.—Man the Only Animal with a
Perfect Hand.—Without the Hand, Man
Could Not Rise Much above the Animals.—
With the Hand, He Constructs, Builds, and
Blesses His Fellows.—With the Hand, He
Smites, Slays, and Injures.—With His Hand
He Pollutes and Degrades Himself.

MY DEAR FRIEND HARRY: At the request of your father I am to continue
these evening Talks for a period, and to-
night I want to call your attention to
some similarity between animals, which
possibly you may not have noticed.

When we speak of animals, you will
remember that man is an animal, although he is the highest in the scale of
being, and God has placed him over all

the other animals. God has endowed him with intellectual powers, so that he can think and reason, has given him a moral sense, so that he might know right from wrong, and has also endowed him with a conscience which approves when he does right and reproves when he does wrong.

Man may pervert his thinking powers, and use them for bad purposes, to devise evil, to plot the injury of his fellow-men, and even to conspire against God. He may also weaken and deaden his moral sense, the same as he does his intellectual powers when he fails to exercise them. These results you see when a boy does not attend school, but neglects to discipline and cultivate his mind; and you also see a similar result when boys and men neglect to attend Sunday-school, the preaching of God's word, and refuse to read good books, or to exercise their moral sense as God has designed it should be exercised and developed. Men may, and many do, turn a deaf ear to conscience by persistently and continuously refusing to obey its dictates, until finally, when conscience reproves they fail, in a large measure, to be conscious of its reproof. The same as when you place an alarm clock in your bedroom and set it for five o'clock in the morning. The first morning when it rings it startles you, and, if you rise immediately and dress, then, morning after morning afterward, when it rings, you will continue to be awakened, so long as you respond to its call. But if, upon the other hand, when the clock rings, you say to yourself that you will sleep "just a moment," and fall into unconsciousness, and sleep until your father or mother awakens you, the next morning when the clock rings you may possibly be wakened, but if you turn over and go to sleep again, after two or three mornings, when the clock rings, you will fail to be aroused at all by its call. So it is with conscience. If we respond to its admonitions all is well; but if we are indifferent when conscience approves or disapproves, after a time we become deaf to its admonitions. Not that conscience fails to reprove, any more than the alarm clock fails to ring; but, having neglected to respond to its

warning, after a time we become indifferent to its reproof, and live on in open
sin as though we had no conscience at
all.

Thus you see that while man is an
animal, he is elevated above all the other
animals by the endowments of intelligence, a moral sense, and a conscience,
which God has given him.

But I desire also to call your attention
to some remarkable similarities and dif-
ferences in the body of man and those
of other animals. Now, if you get down
upon your hands and knees upon the
floor, you will notice that there is a great
likeness in the form of your body and
the form of the body of a horse, or cow,
or dog, and all four-footed animals.
When in this position you will see that
your arms and hands, in a large measure,
correspond to their forelegs and feet.
In some, as with the dog and cat, the
small extensions, or toes on their feet,
correspond also with the fingers and toes
upon your hands and feet. With others,
as in the case of the horse, the fingers
and toes are gathered into one foot, and
the nails, which are on the ends of your

fingers and toes are enlarged and gathered into one thick nail, which forms the hoof of the horse, or the double hoof of the cow.

Now if you stand on your feet, and pass your arms behind you, and hold them pretty well up on your back, you will see that the form of your body in that position resembles the form of the body of a bird; your legs and feet corresponding to their legs and feet, and your arms corresponding to their wings. The study of such similarities learned men call the study of comparative anatomy. So you see that there is some similarity between the construction of our bodies and the construction of the bodies of other animals.

But there is one particular in which the human body differs from all the others. Man is the only animal to whom God has given a perfect hand. Even with our intellectual endowment, if God had not given us our hands it would have been physically impossible for man to have risen much above the level of the lower animals, but with his hands man prepares his food, compounds his medicine, manufactures his clothing, builds houses in which to live, writes books, prints papers, constructs all kinds of machinery, builds railroads and great steamships with which he can outdo even the birds in their flight. With all these things God is doubtless well pleased.

But because of the evil in man's mind and the wickedness in his heart he also uses his hands to inflict pain and injury upon his fellow-man. He constructs great cannons, and gunboats, and other instruments of death with which he destroys his fellow-man in battle. Moved by the wickedness in his heart, and encouraged and helped on by Satan and others who are wicked like himself, man uses his hands to accomplish many things which are very displeasing in the sight of God.

But, strange to say, man is possibly the only animal which persistently pollutes and degrades his own body, and this would not have been easily possible to him if God had not given him hands, which He designed should prove useful and a means of great help and blessing to him in his life upon the earth.

In order that the hand might not be used for degrading his own body, or for the injury of his fellow-men, God endowed man with wisdom, with a moral sense, and with conscience, so that his hands should be to him a source of help and blessing, and not a means of defilement and injury and thus prove a curse.

CYLINDER IX.

MY DEAR FRIEND HARRY: When God gave man hands, He also gave him intelligence, a moral sense, and a conscience that he might use them aright. With his hands God meant that man should lift himself up infinitely above the animals, but some men, and we are sorry to say boys, too, use their hands so as to debase themselves below the level of the most degraded brute. Instead of using their hands as intelligent and moral beings should do, they use their hands so as to pollute their bodies, by handling and toying with their sexual member in such a way as to produce a sensation, or feeling, which may give a momentary pleasure, but which results in the most serious of injuries to the moral, intellectual, and physical powers. God did not give us a sexual member or organ to be used in this way, and such a use of it is called self-pollution or masturbation.

Man is the only animal except one whose sexual organ is exposed on the outside of his body, and the only animal to whom self-pollution is mechanically or physically possible. The rare instances which are in conflict with this statement are accidental and altogether exceptional. In the care and use of the sexual member God has reposed the greatest trust in man's intelligence and moral sense. Upon no other animal has God placed such confidence and responsibilities as upon man. But because of the wickedness of the human heart, the temptations of Satan, and sometimes also because of ignorance upon this important subject, even young boys begin to go wrong, and with no one to instruct and warn them, they pursue evil habits which result in great injury, and

if the practice is not stopped the individual is plunged into great vice and
degradation.

I wish that I might say to you, Harry,
that but very few boys have ever known
anything of this vice, but I do not believe that such a statement would be
true. I can say, however, that many
pure-minded and innocent boys have
learned the habit in very innocent ways,
and in the beginning not even mistrust-
ing that the habit was either wicked or
injurious. Many boys at a very early
age have discovered the sensation by
sliding down the banisters, or at a little
later period in life by climbing and de-
scending trees, by riding on horse-back,
and some because of uncleanness of the
sexual member have experienced an
itching of these parts, and when relief
has been sought by chafing or rubbing,
the child has been introduced to the
habit of self-pollution. Sometimes by
constipation of the bowels, or in simpler
language, a failure to go regularly each
morning and pass from the lower portion
of the body the worn out and waste
matter which has accumulated in the in-

testines, and this neglect, when often repeated or long continued, results in
producing what is called constipation,
which often proves very injurious, and,
for causes that I need not now stop to
explain, produces a tendency to local
sensitiveness and leads to self-pollution.

A similar, or even greater sensitiveness of the sexual member is sometimes
produced by pin-worms in the rectum, or
lowest part of the intestines. But I am
sorry also to say that masturbation is
sometimes even taught by one boy to
another, and during the infancy of children, even nurses, sometimes, in ignorance of the terrible evil and sad consequences of their act, practice this
destructive habit upon very young children for the purpose of diverting their
thoughts, so that they will not cry, or
in order that they may be quieted and
fall asleep. It is terrible to think that
intelligent people could do such things,
but on account of the prevalence of these
practices it is necessary that we should
understand the danger to which children
are exposed so that we may be properly
upon our guard against the temptations

from without and, by the aid of our intelligence, be saved from the terrible consequences which are visited upon many because of the evil practices which they begin in their ignorance.

I trust, my dear boy, that you may be saved from this and all other forms of vice.

CYLINDER X.

The Sexual Member a Part of the Reproductive System. — The Reproductive System Defined.—Illustrated By a Watch.—The Different Parts of the Digestive System.— God Gave Us a Reproductive System for the Wisest and Most Beneficent Ends.—By Wrong Thoughts of Them, We Dishonor God.—To Be Held in Purity and Honor.— Our Bodies the Temples of the Holy Ghost. —The Holy Place, and the Holy of Holies.— The Wonderful Mystery of Creative Power. —How the Mind, Imagination, and Heart Are Polluted.—What the Bible Says Upon These Subjects.

MY DEAR FRIEND HARRY: Last night I told you how some young boys, and older boys also, pollute and degrade their own bodies by unnecessarily and injuriously handling or scratching and chafing the sexual member. God gave us this member to serve us in the removal of the wasted or worn out fluids of the body, and also made it one of the parts of the human reproductive system.

What the reproductive system or organs are to plants I told you on a previous cylinder. They are the organs in the male, and also in the female plant which are engaged in the production of the seeds from which life is to be reproduced. Something of the nature and office of the reproductive system may be learned by supposing that a watch could be built and given power to keep its own wheels, and all its works in repair, so that it would not have to be taken to the jeweler's to have any worn parts replaced by new parts. Then suppose that in addition to this renewing power it should also be endowed with a power to reproduce other watches; so that while it was keeping accurate time, renewing its own wear and wasting of the wheels and all the parts, it should also have the power to produce other watches; little baby watches, which should also have imparted to them the power to grow and, when they became fully grown and were large watches, then also in turn, from time to time, they also should produce other watches. This new power by which the watch would produce

others would be called the reproductive
power, and if there were certain parts in
the watch which were devoted wholly to
the production of these little baby
watches, such portions of the watch
would together be called the reproductive organs.

Now the sexual member is only one
part of the reproductive system: the
same, as in our bodies, we have a digestive system composed of several members or parts. The food is taken into the
mouth and, after being chewed or masti-
cated, as we say, is passed into the
stomach, where it undergoes changes
which fit it to be received by the intestines, so that it may be converted into
blood, and thus strengthen the body and
maintain life. Now the mouth, the pas-
sage-way into the stomach, and such
portions of the intestines as are engaged
in the work of digesting and preparing
the food for use in the blood—all these
different members together constitute
the digestive system. So the sexual
member is one portion of the reproductive system, and the other portions in
men are partly without the body and

partly within the body. So, when taken together, we speak of the sexual organs and their functions as the reproductive system, and this portion of our body has been created by God Himself for the wisest and most beneficent ends. Sometimes boys think of their sexual parts in a very low and degraded way, and thus greatly dishonor God and wrong themselves. Whatever God has created deserves to be held in honor and esteem. God has endowed us with no holier or more sacred duty than that of reproducing our species, and we should receive and accept this high and holy office from the hands of our infinite Creator with reverence, and maintain these members of our body in purity and honor. Dr. Sperry, a Christian physician, says " The propagation of our species is the highest, the divinest act of our physical life." And no man, with a pure heart and a thoughtful mind, can come to any other conclusion.

I am glad, my dear friend Harry, that your parents often study the Bible with you, that they may make its truths plain to your mind. It is therefore very

proper in talking with you to-night upon
this subject of self-pollution, that I
should refer you to First Corinthians,
sixth chapter, eighteenth and nineteenth
verses, where Paul, in writing upon this
very subject, says, "Flee fornification.
. . He that committeth fornication sin-
neth against his own body. What?
Know ye not that your body is the temple of the Holy Ghost which is in you?"
Now the Temple at Jerusalem was one
of the most sacred buildings in all the
world. The entire structure was sacred,
but within the building there was a place
called "The Holy Place," and in the interior of that Holy Place there was a
still more sacred inclosure called "The
Holy of Holies." Here dwelt the un-
approachable divine presence, and toward this Holy of Holies the Israelites
throughout the entire nation and
throughout the world, never turned their
faces but in devout reverence. So our
entire bodies are holy, and are to be
held in perpetual honor, but I am sure
that no thoughtful person can properly
study this subject of the human body
without thinking of the reproductive sys-

tem as the holy of holies in which God dwells within us in the wonderful mystery of reproductive power.

Before saying good-night to you I want to remind you that the body may not only be outwardly polluted by the hands, but the mind, the imagination, and the heart may be polluted by means of the eye when we look upon improper things and upon indecent pictures; and we may also produce the same bad results with the ear, by listening to vile stories, bad words, and evil suggestions. The eye and the ear are gateways into our minds and hearts, and we should guard them with great care. These are some of the avenues by which the sacred temple of our bodies is entered by evil influences, and we should remember that the Bible also says in First Corinthians, third chapter and nineteenth verse, " If any man defile the temple of God, him shall God destroy." I am sure that you do not desire to be banished from the presence of God, and therefore you should also remember what it says in another place (Matthew v. 8):

" Blessed are the pure in heart, for they shall see God."

To-morrow night I shall tell you what are the consequences in boys of the misuse of these reproductive organs.

PART III.

What are the Consequences in Boys of the Abuse
of the Reproductive Organs.

CYLINDER XI.

MY DEAR FRIEND HARRY: No boy
can toy with the exposed portions of his
reproductive system without finally suffering very serious consequences. In
the beginning it may seem to a boy a
trifling matter, and yet from the very
first his conscience will tell him that he
is doing something that is very wrong.
It is on this account that a boy who
yields to such an evil temptation will
seek a secluded, solitary place, and it is
because of this fact that it is called the
" solitary vice." Because the entire be-

ing of the one who indulges in this practice is debased and polluted by his own personal act it is also called "self-pollution." It is also called "Onanism," because, for a similar offense, nearly four thousand years ago, God punished Onan with death (Genesis xxxviii. 3--10). This sin is also known by another name, and is called "masturbation," a word which is made from two Latin words which mean "To pollute by the hand."

Each of these words tells something of the vile character of this sin. But words are scarcely capable of describing the dreadful consequences which are suffered by those who persist in this practice. I do not believe, my dear friend Harry, that you have become a victim of this destructive vice, and I would be glad to believe that you have never accidentally learned or have been deliberately taught to engage in it. Knowing, however, the dangers to which, like all boys, you are exposed, and also appreciating the fact that intellectual boys, because of a more highly wrought nervous organization and because of keener sensibilities, are much more liable to become addicted to this vice than boys of a lower grade of intellect and with less sensitive bodies, I regard it important that you should be as intelligent and well informed upon this subject as upon any other. This is necessary so that, by knowing in advance the character and consequences of such a course, you may avoid the evil into which even men, as late in life as twenty-five and thirty years of age, sometimes fall because of ignorance. In this as in other things, " To be forewarned is to be forearmed." Every young boy should be properly informed upon this subject, for even those who may be safely guarded from defilement of thought and life from outward influences are nevertheless exposed to those inward physical conditions which may produce local irritation and disease, and where such a diseased condition is ignorantly permitted to continue, masturbation soon becomes a fixed habit, and is likely to be practiced with such violence that idiocy, and even death, may, and often does come speedily. Nothing so much favors the continuance and spread of this awful vice as ignorance, and only by being early and purely taught on this important subject can the coming boys and men be saved from the awful consequences which are ruining morally, mentally, and physically thousands of boys every year.

As I have already said, one of the first things which a boy does who undertakes to practice this vice is to seek solitude. From the very first his conscience disapproves, and so he cannot engage in the evil which he proposes to himself without violating his moral sense. Indeed, his moral nature is the first to suffer. This, my dear boy, is an important fact, and if you were ever to fall a victim to this vice, you would find that even with the first sense of guilt there would come a spirit of rebellion against God and against your parents. You would soon begin to call into question the wisdom and goodness of God. Your pleasure in good books, in religious instruction, in the Sunday-school, the Bible, the Church, and all holy things would rapidly diminish. You would soon find in your heart a rebellious feel-

ing which would lead you to be disobedient, cross, irritable, and reproachful.
You would begin to lose faith in all that
is good, and as you persisted in your
sin, you would grow less and less like
Jesus and more and more like Satan.
In other words the moral nature is the
first to suffer from sexual vice, and
whenever you hear a boy or man boasting of his doubts and railing against
God, against the Bible, against purity
and virtue, you may rest assured that this
feeling grows out of some solitary or
social, some secret or open sin or vice
which has affected his moral nature, and
is degrading and debasing his heart.

If this effect upon the moral nature
were the only result of this solitary vice,
the consequences would be sufficient to
turn any intelligent and thoughtful boy
from the practice. But its effects upon
the mind and body are also of the most
serious nature, and of these I will speak
to you to-morrow night.

CYLINDER XII.

Effect on the Character of Boys.—After the Effects upon the Moral Nature, Those of the Nervous System Appear.—The Spasm of the Nerves.—The Mind Next to Suffer.—The Visible Effects upon the Mind.—Physical Effects Follow.—Character of These Effects Stated.—Competent Physician Can Judge Accurately.—The Habit Grows Strong, and the Will Grows Weak.—Results Where the Practice Is Persisted in.—The Treatment in Extreme Cases.—The Importance of Early Instruction.

MY DEAR FRIEND HARRY: If I had time there are many things I would like to tell you concerning the way in which the effects of vice are manifested upon the moral nature and are seen in the lives of sinning boys and men; but I must hasten on, lest you weary.

After great changes have been effected in the boy's character, and the bright, frank, happy, and obedient boy has become the fretful, irritable, stolid, and reticent boy, and when he can no longer

look people squarely and frankly in the
face, but seeks to avoid meeting people,
pulls his cap down so as to hide his eyes,
and goes about with a shy and guilty
bearing, then changes which are mental
and physical may be confidently expected.

After the moral nature, the nervous
system is the next to suffer. In no other
portion of the human body are so large
a number of nerves brought so closely
together as in the reproductive organ.
In the act of masturbation, these nerves
are wrought upon in such a manner as
to produce most serious results. The
pleasurable emotion with which the beginning is attended culminates in a
spasm of the nerves, terminating for the
time all pleasure, and leaving the nerves
as wasted and depleted as the body of a
person whose entire physical system has
been brought under the influence of a
spasm, or fit as it is called. You will
easily understand how such violent
shocks to these special nerves are com-
municated to the nerves throughout the
entire body, and if such shocks are repeated, or long continued, the entire

nervous system will become shattered and ruined beyond all hope of complete recovery.

While the nerves are thus being ruined, the mind is also suffering. The bright boy that stood at the head of the class is losing his power to comprehend and retain his lessons. His memory fails him. His mind begins to lack grasp and grip. He cannot, as formerly, take hold and hold fast. Gradually he loses his place and sinks to the foot of his class. He is no longer positive and self-reliant. He no longer has his accustomed pleasure in the vigorous romp, the hearty laugh, and good fellowship which characterize a boy with a vigorous mind and a strong body.

While these moral and mental changes are taking place, the physical effects do not stop with the nerves. The health declines. The eyes lose their luster. The skin becomes sallow. The muscles become flabby. There is an unnatural languor. Every little effort is followed by weariness. There is a great indifference to exertion. Work becomes distasteful and irksome. He complains of pain in the back; of headache and dizziness. The hands become cold and clammy. The digestion becomes poor, the appetite fitful. The heart palpitates. He sits in a stooping position, becomes hollow-chested, and the entire body, instead of enlarging into a strong, manly, frame, becomes wasted, and many signs give promise of early decline and death.

These, my dear friend Harry, are some of the more prominent symptoms and effects of masturbation in boys and young men when the habit is frequently indulged, or after being continued for a period. Some of these conditions, it is true, may be produced by other forms of bodily disease, and on that account the unskilled are likely to misjudge, but a competent physician ought, at all times, to be able to judge accurately in any given case of the cause, or causes, which have produced such results.

One serious difficulty with all who become addicted to this terrible and destructive vice is that, while the body, mind, and moral character become weak, the habit becomes strong. The will itself may become so weak that even when the person is told of the destructive nature and sad consequences of the vice, he may not even desire to discontinue the practice, nor even really desire to escape the fearful consequences which are sure to come later on; and even where there is sufficient manhood and character left to desire to be free, the will is often so weak as to require a fierce struggle for a long period.

You will see, from what I have said, that this secret vice is attended with most serious consequences. But I have not yet told you the worst. If persisted in, masturbation will not only undermine, but completely overthrow the health. If the body is naturally strong, the mind may give way first, and in extreme cases imbecility and insanity may, and often do come as the inevitable result. Where the body is not naturally strong, a general wasting may be followed by consumption, or life may be terminated by any one of many diseases.

The terrible and helpless condition of those upon whom this habit has permanently fastened itself, you may be able to judge from the fact that, in order to

prevent the repetition of the act of masturbation, and if possible permanently to
cure the victim of this vice, boys often
have to be put in a "strait-jacket,"
sometimes have their hands fastened behind their backs, sometimes their hands
are tied to the posts of the bed, or fastened by ropes or chains to rings in the
wall; and in various other ways extreme
measures have to be resorted to in the
effort to save the individual from total
mental and physical self-destruction.
And I am sorry to say that even these
extreme measures are not always suc-
cessful in restraining the individual or
effecting a cure.

I think you will see, my dear boy, how
important it is that all boys should be
duly warned, and in good time also, of
the terrible results of this destructive
vice. You will understand why your
own dear Papa should have asked me to
continue and send you further Talks in
the phonograph, after I had answered
you the question which you asked of
your Mamma, and which, because of her
sickness, I had the honor of being asked
to tell you. Your parents are too intelli-

gent, and love you too much, to be indifferent to the importance of these serious questions. They have not been willing that, on account of ignorance, you should be exposed to those terrible dangers, and as this knowledge is imparted to you, and as you come to know of the sad results of the sins into which many previously pure-minded and well-meaning boys have fallen through ignorance, you should thank God for the intelligent love of your parents, and for His kind providence, by which you have been kept from this prevalent and destructive vice.

Recognizing what your parents have desired for you in this matter, it will be very proper that to-morrow night I should remind you what injustice would be done them and others, if you were ever to become addicted to sexual vice, in this or any other form.

CYLINDER XIII.

The Boy who Practices Solitary Vice Not the
Solitary Sufferer.—The Sins of Children
Visited upon Their Parents.—Parents often
the Greatest Sufferers.—What Parents Do
for Their Children.—During Infancy.—Dur-
ing Childhood.—Should Not Disappoint
Their Hopes.—Brothers and Sisters Made to
Suffer.—His Children after Him Must Suffer
the Results of His Sin.—We Reproduce Our-
selves.—Cannot Transmit what We Do Not
Possess.—What We Are That Our Children
Will Be.—The Character of the Boys and
Girls of To-day Determines the Character of
the Nation a Hundred Years to Come.

MY DEAR FRIEND HARRY: From
what I told you last night and the night
before you will understand something of
the sad consequences of solitary vice; yet
the boy himself is not the solitary, or
only sufferer.   No one can do wrong in
any way without causing that others
must also bear, at least in some measure,
the results of his sin.   Not only are the
sins of the parents visited upon the chil-

dren, but the sins of the children are also visited upon the parents.

If by your own act you were to impair your health, enfeeble your intellect, and destroy your usefulness, it is a question whether your parents might not be as great or even greater sufferers than yourself. Think for a moment of what your own parents have done for you. After Mamma had brought you into the world at the risk of her own life, and at the cost of much pain and suffering, for months she gave herself almost wholly to nourishing and caring for you. When the various sicknesses peculiar to childhood came, she guarded you carefully lest you should take cold and die, or be left with impaired sight or hearing, or in some other way be caused to suffer during the remainder of your life with some physical infirmity. When you had the scarlet fever, for days and weeks Mamma and Papa gave themselves almost constantly to you. Day and night they watched over you, and for months, for fear of catching this dreadful disease, or communicating it to others, no one came to the house; and for your sake they cheerfully watched and suffered all without complaint.

Ever since you were born, they have been laboring to provide you every comfort. They have been careful about your instruction and education. They have guarded you from evil companions and dangerous influences of every sort, and I am sure you will readily see what a disappointment and sorrow it would be to them, if you were to do wrong. What a sorrow to Papa and Mamma it would be to see their boy with sallow face, glassy eye, drooping form, without energy, force, or purpose, a laggard in school, shy, avoiding the society of others, disliking good books, avoiding the Sunday-school, and desiring to escape from every elevating Christian influence. Nothing I am sure would bring greater pain to the hearts of Papa and Mamma, than to know that their dear boy, whom they hoped to prepare for great usefulness, had turned aside into ways of sin and evil which were surely disappointing all their hopes and ruining their boy, both for this world and the world to come.

Not only to them, but what a sorrow and regret would come to that little baby sister when she should grow to womanhood, and then, when she should justly be proud to turn to you for counsel, sympathy, and help, be humiliated to find that you were weak, nervous, and unworthy of the respect and love which she would under other conditions have been glad to have bestowed upon you. Not only would you be wronging your own sister, but you would also be wronging that pure, sweet girl, whom, in the providence of God, we may rightly trust is being prepared to crown and bless your manhood, and with whom you cannot expect to be honored and happy unless your life has been characterized by the same purity and honor which you shall have a right to expect of her.

But the consequences which result from masturbation do not stop with the boy who practices it, nor with his parents, brothers and sisters, friends and relatives, but where such a boy lives to become a man, if he marries, and should become a father, his children after him must suffer to some degree the results of his sin. If his life has disqualified him for thrift, and his children on this account are born in poverty, this would be one of the results which they would suffer. But if his physical powers have been impaired by vice, or any other cause, he cannot transmit perfect physical, mental, and moral powers to his children. For neither physically nor financially can a man transmit or give to his children that which he does not himself possess. As in grain so in human life, if the quality of the grain which is sown in the field is poor, the grain that grows from it will be inferior. When a boy injures his reproductive powers, so that when a man his sexual secretion shall be of an inferior quality, his offspring will show it in their physical, mental, and moral natures. So you see that even a young boy may prepare the way to visit upon his children that are to be, the results of vices and sins committed long years before they were born. This surely is a very impressive thought, and you will see how even the little boys of to-day are unconsciously molding and shaping not only the character and destiny of the children that are to come after them, but how they are also shaping the history and destiny of the nation. The thought and conduct, the aspirations and ambitions of the boys and girls in the kindergartens and primary schools are to-day cultivating and developing in them that life and character which will determine what shall be the dominant characteristics of this nation a hundred years to come.

I would that every boy in the land might know these facts, so that he might intelligently resolve to take such care of his health that his children might be blessed with vigorous bodies; that he would so exercise his mind that his children might inherit added capacity to acquire knowledge; and that he would so obey the laws of morality that his children might inherit a tend toward virtue, uprighteousness, and religion.

You see, then, how important it is that nothing should be done that will weaken any of the faculties or powers which God has given you, and to-morrow night I will endeavor to tell you briefly how boys may preserve their entire bodies in purity and strength.

PART IV.

How Boys may Preserve their Entire Bodies in
Purity and Strength.

CYLINDER XIV.

How Purity and Strength May Be Preserved.—
Our Space Not Sufficient to Tell All.—
Subject to Be Pursued in other Books.—
" Cleanliness Next to Godliness."—Purity of
Mind and Body.—A Pure Heart the First Re-
quisite.—Guarding the Heart.—Danger from
Impure Books.—Purity of the Body.—The
Weekly and Daily Bath. — The Rite of
Circumcision as Related to Purity.—Not only
the External, but also the Internal Portions
of the Body to Be Kept Pure.—Emptying
out of Waste Fluids and Solids.—The Lesson
Taught by the Fire in the Grate and Stove.—
The Fire, or Combustion, in our Bodies.—
Smoke and Perspiration.—Ashes and Waste
Substances in the Body.—Importance of
Emptying Waste Pipes of the Body
Regularly.

MY DEAR FRIEND HARRY: I prom-
ised to attempt to tell you to-night how
boys may preserve their entire bodies in
purity and strength.

In talking to a boy who has been
blessed with parents as intelligent and
judicious as your Papa and Mamma, I
cannot hope that all, or even much that

I shall say will be entirely new. I may hope, however, to emphasize by repetition what your parents have told you, and thus by "Line upon line, and precept upon precept" confirm and deepen the impression of duties and rules which may now seem very simple, but which in later years you will recognize as both important and valuable. To tell you all that might be desirable upon this subject would require that we should consider it together each night for several weeks. We can, however, only give three or four evenings to this topic, and I hope that later on you will pursue it further, by reading some valuable books upon the subject.*   I shall try, however, to give you the largest amount of information in the shortest time and simplest way.

You have doubtless often heard it said that, "Cleanliness is next to Godliness." True cleanliness includes purity,

* The author would recommend such books as "The Marvels of our Bodily Dwelling," by Mrs. Mary Wood-Allen, M. D.   Parents should place in the hands of their children the best books of this class.

both of body and mind. If immodest
and impure thoughts are permitted to
dwell in the mind, they will soon work
themselves out in the life. The Bible
says of man, "As he thinketh in his
heart, so is he." Thought soon becomes life and character. You see,
then, that it is important that we keep
our minds and our thoughts pure.

The most important requisite in se-
curing and keeping a pure mind is to
have a pure heart, and God alone can
give you a pure heart, and our prayer
should be "Create in me a clean heart,
O God; and renew a right spirit within
me" (Psalm li. 10). The Bible says,
"Blessed are the pure in heart, for
they shall see God" (Matthew v. 8).
If you have not yet given your heart
fully to the Saviour, that truly is your
first duty and your only safety and salvation. When you have this pure heart
which God alone can give, it is your
duty to guard it well. For the Bible's
injunction is, "Keep thy heart with all
diligence; for out of it are the issues of
life" (Proverbs iv. 23).

That you may properly guard your

heart, you will need to avoid with great care all books which are immodest or impure. Many, very many books are evil and impure in character, and not a few are so in purpose. Never read, handle, or listen to a book or paper which you might not ask your Mamma or Papa to read aloud with you. In all these matters, make your parents your counselors and protectors. Turn away in disgust from those who would pollute your mind with vile stories or immodest conversation. For your companions and associates, choose only the pure and the good. If such could not be found, it were better to abide alone. It would be much easier for a bad companion to pull you down than for you to lift him up.

Not only the mind, but the body should be kept pure and clean. Every person should bathe his entire body at least once each week, and twice a week is still better. When a boy, I began to take a hand bath in cold water each morning before dressing. This soon grew into a fixed habit, and has been continued throughout my life with great physical benefit. If begun in the summer, there will be no danger of taking cold, and when the cold water and weather of the winter come, the bath will be followed by a warm glow and much invigoration. After a good rubbing with a coarse towel, the hands should be used to rub the entire body vigorously.

To insure the cleanliness of the sexual member, and thus the more effectually secure purity, and strengthen virtue among His chosen people, God instituted the rite of circumcision, which was performed when the male child was eight days old. This rite consisted in drawing forward and cutting off the loose skin at the end of the sexual member. In this way it became easier for the parent, and later for the child, to keep the glans, or end of the sexual member free from the smegma, or soapy substance that is liable to gather under the foreskin, and which, if not removed, will in a few days set up an irritation, and render the child an easy subject of sexual excitement and masturbation. When taking your regular weekly bath, it is always well to draw the foreskin back gently and cleanse carefully that portion of the sexual member. This act of cleansing should be done conscientiously and religiously, avoiding any act which would pollute the mind or degrade the body.

Not only the exterior, but the interior of the body also is to be kept pure by being kept clean. The largest part of the impurity which is to be washed from the exterior of the body consists of the worn out and wasted fluids and solids which are passed out of the body through the pores of the skin, mostly in the form of perspiration. Frequent bathing is necessary to keep the pores open, so that the body may be kept in good health. But a large accumulation of waste matter, both in the form of fluids and solids, is also cast out of the body in bulk, or in considerable quantities, at a single time.

How we come to have these waste substances in the body, perhaps you will best understand by noticing the burning of the fire in the grate or stove. The burning of the wood and coal produces

heat, and if the fire is to be kept burning, fuel must be added from time to
time. As the fuel burns away, ashes
accumulate. A small quantity passes
up the chimney in the form of smoke,
and that which remains in the form of
ashes must be removed or the grate will
be clogged up, the draught cut off, and
the fire go out. The same is true of our
bodies. The warmth of our bodies is
caused by the changes effected in the
lungs, liver, and muscles, by the processes of life, which in many ways closely
resemble the burning of fuel in the
stove. That part which passes off
through the pores in perspiration resembles that portion of the ashes which
passes up the chimney in the form of
smoke, and that which accumulates as
fluids and solids in those portions of our
bodies which God has provided for their
reception, correspond to the ashes which
gather in the ash pan under the grate.
Now, if the ash pan is not emptied daily,
the ashes will pile up until they clog
the grate, cut off the draught, and put
out the fire. And in like manner, if the
bladder and rectum are not emptied at

proper intervals, the entire interior of the body will be stopped up, all the offices of the body will be hindered, these offensive substances will be clogged and retained in the blood, the brain and all portions of the body will feel dull and heavy, and if long continued or often repeated, sickness and disease will surely 'follow.

If you desire to be strong and well, empty the waste pipes of the body regularly and faithfully. The waste fluid should always be wholly emptied out the last thing before getting into the bed at night, upon rising in the morning, and at intervals of from four to six hours throughout the day. The waste solids should be emptied from the body with unfailing regularity each day, and the great mass of cleanly and careful people have found it best to make this the first duty each morning immediately after breakfast. Without care and regularity in performing these two duties, good health, a vigorous body, and a clean mind are altogether impossible. In order that the inhabitants of a house may be comfortable and happy, it is not enough that the outside of the house should be nicely painted, but the inside of the house must be cleanly and pure. To be healthy and happy, keep your body clean and pure, both without and within.

CYLINDER XV.

Slow Oxidation, Called Rusting; Rapid, Called
Burning.—Best of Fuel for the Fire in Our
Bodies.—Choice and Preparation of Food.—
Discover what Foods Do Not Agree with
You. — Abnormal   Appetites. — What   to
Drink.—Danger of All Stimulants.—The
Ruin Caused by Intoxicating Liquors.—The
Dangerous Cigarette.—Tobacco Universally
and Seriously Injurious to Young Boys.—
Effect upon the Brain.—Upon the Body.—
Upon the Reproductive Organs.

MY DEAR FRIEND HARRY: Last
night I spoke to you of the warmth and
changes which take place in our bodies
under the figure of a fire in the grate or
stove. In very many respects the similarity is more of a fact than a figure.
In our bodies, the combustion, or oxidation, or burning, is slower, but none
the less real. When such oxidation, or
burning, is slow, as in the gradual destruction of iron which is exposed to the
weather, we call it rusting; when it pro-

ceeds rapidly, as with coal and wood, it is called burning. The process in both instances, however, is the same. In the human body the burning is not so rapid as with wood, but much more rapid than the oxidation of iron. The Bible recognizes this scientific fact where it speaks of death as a light, a candle, or a lamp. In the book of Job (xviii. 5) it says, "The light of the wicked shall be put out," and in Proverbs (xxiv. 20), "The candle of the wicked shall be put out," and in another chapter (xiii. 9), "The lamp of the wicked shall be put out."

Since the important changes that take place in our bodies so closely resemble the combustion of wood and coal, it is very proper that we should inquire into what kind of fuel should be used to keep this flame of our physical life burning most successfully and with the best result.

There are so many kinds of food that it will be impossible to speak of any of them separately. Never eat any but the most wholesome foods. These should be properly cooked, eaten in proper quantities, in sufficient varieties, and at

regular intervals. Always observe carefully the effects of what you eat. If you
have a headache, a fever, or even when
you feel cross and irritable, inquire carefully into the character and quantity of
what you ate from twelve to forty-eight
hours previously, and in this way, by
observation and thoughtfulness, you
will make many valuable discoveries
concerning your own well-being and
health. Study thoughtfully the many
rules of health prepared by others,
always remembering, however, that any
slight modification to suit your own best
needs will be dependent upon your careful observation and study of your own
body. Never eat anything that dis-
agrees with you simply because it tastes
good. Do not live solely that you may
eat, but eat solely that you may live.

Some boys, and girls, too, weaken
and disease their bodies by cultivating
and developing an unnatural appetite
for vinegar, salt, cloves, coffee, slate
pencils, and other substances which are
taken in such form and in such quantities as to become very injurious in many
ways. Such habits, if not early aban-

doned, lead to secret and social vice, prepare the individual for intemperance, and pave the way for permanent injury, or even for total wreck and ruin. The sad effects of such a course we have ourselves witnessed in the lives of several who were boys and girls with us years ago.

What is true of eating is true also of drinking. Drink only that which confers good health. Pure water, at the temperature it flows from the spring, is the best form of drink for both young and old. The boy who drinks tea and coffee while he is growing can never grow to be as large, muscular, and manly a man as he would become if he drank only good, pure water. Tea and coffee are stimulants, and these can never be taken during the growing years without lessening the vitality, strength, and growth.

As you value your health, happiness, usefulness, and even life itself, never take intoxicating liquors in any form. Look about you and see the ruin caused by rum in the lives of others. Learn lessons of wisdom by thoughtful observation, rather than by sad experience, and remember the true teachings of the Bible on this subject: " Wine is a mocker, strong drink is raging; and whosoever is deceived thereby is not wise " (Proverbs xx. 1). It also says of wine and strong drink, what you may also see about you, if you are observant, " At the last it biteth like a serpent, and stingeth like an adder " (Proverbs xxiii. 32).

What I have said of tea and coffee is true also of the effect of tobacco, only to a much greater degree. The cigarette is small, looks harmless, and therefore presents to boys one of the most dangerous and destructive forms of temptation. It may be possible that some few men, who have passed their thirtieth birthday, whose bodies are fully matured, and whose physical and mental habit is naturally sluggish and heavy, may smoke tobacco in moderation without seeming injurious effects, but it is absolutely certain that no growing boy can use tobacco in any form without positive, immediate, and permanent injury. Look carefully at the boys you

meet who use cigarettes. In proportion
as they are addicted to the cigarette,
they are stunted and dwarfed in their
muscular development. If you can suc-
ceed in finding a single boy, who
smokes cigarettes in any considerable
quantity, whose muscles are well developed and firm, whose skin is not sallow,
the white of whose eyes is not clouded
and the surface glassy, you will have
discovered what many careful observers
among men have failed to find. Tobacco always stunts and dwarfs a growing boy, and the effect upon the brain is
as marked and serious as upon the body.
In the schools and colleges careful
observation has demonstrated that those
who use tobacco in any form fall much
below the average standing of those in
the same classes who do not use tobacco
at all. The carefully recorded development in height, weight, and intellectual
capacity of students during the four
years spent in our colleges, shows that
those who do not smoke gain in weight
twenty-four per cent. more than those in
the same classes who do smoke, in
height, thirty-seven per cent. more, and

in the size of the chest, forty-two per cent more. What is true in the colleges is even more marked, although less noticed by actual test, in all the primary and preparatory schools throughout the land.

The use of tobacco seriously affects the powers of the brain, the health of every organ of the body, and especially the healthy and vigorous growth of the reproductive system. If the injurious effects which come as the result of smoking or chewing tobacco were limited to the individual who uses it, the consequences would not be so bad, but when we remember that, " We are not separate units, but are links in a living chain of endless transmission," we see how any injury done to our own bodies must be transmitted to the children that come after us. As I told you some evenings previous, what you are that your children will most easily and most naturally become, and what you would have them to be, that, even in your growing years, you must yourself seek to be. Smoking is not only injurious, but expensive, and is also attended with numerous dangers.

I had hoped to include in my Talk to-night some subjects which we shall be compelled to leave until to-morrow night. Till then, think on these things.

CYLINDER XVI.

God Intended Man to Work.—Many Seem to
Be Born Lazy.—All Must Learn to Work.—
Some Forms of Labor Call into Service only
a Few Muscles.—Every Muscle Should Do
Service. — Importance of Exercise. — The
Boy's Bible and Dumb-Bells.—The Muscles
Developed by Exercise.—This Not True of
the Sexual Member.—Importance of Recrea-
tion.—Difference between Exercise and
Recreation.—This Illustrated.—So much of
Zest and Pleasure May Be Put into Daily
Duty as to Convert it into Recreation.—
Daily Food and Daily Exercise.—Importance
of Sufficient Sleep.—The Best Hours for
Sleep.

MY DEAR FRIEND HARRY: Purity
and strength of body and mind cannot
be maintained simply by eating the best
and most nourishing kinds of food.
God has made our bodies in such a way
that if we would be strong, healthy, and
happy, we must also work. Even before the Fall, God gave Adam and Eve
something to do. This was necessary

for both their health and their happiness.
They were not to spend their time in
idleness. They were put in the garden of
Eden " To dress it and to keep it." By
nature, at first, none of us like to work.
We all seem to be born lazy, but we
must be taught to work, and should be
put at it and kept at it, at such intervals
as are best suited to teach us the art, and
enable us to acquire the taste for work.
Do not shrink from doing the many
little things which are asked of you.
Be faithful to every duty, in school and
out of it. And remember the old and
valuable self-evident truth, "Whatsoever
is worth doing at all is worth doing
well, and if it is not worth doing well,
it is not worth doing at all." Never be
ashamed of honest toil. Dignify your
work by doing it well, and you will be
honored and blessed in the doing of it.

Some kinds of toil tax the mind rather
than the body. Some other kinds tax
only a few muscles of the body, and
leave all the others unused. In order
that the blood may circulate freely to
every muscle, and that the entire body
may be kept strong, it is important that

every muscle in the body should be called into service. To secure this, nearly all persons need exercise. What kind it should be must be determined by the character of the daily occupation. The boy who has walked in the furrow or followed the harrow all day will not need in the evening to take a walk for exercise. He might enjoy a row on the lake, or a swim in the stream, or he might be rested and benefited by such a change of labor as would call into service an entirely different set of muscles. If he were to change to the seat on the corn planter, the reaper, or the horse rake, he would rest one set of tired muscles while another set were doing duty, and, by a simple change of work, find the needed rest.

There are but few kinds of work which call all the muscles into service, and therefore, to wake up the unused powers and keep the entire body strong and well, all classes of people can be greatly benefited by some judicious form of exercise. Whenever I go into a boy's room, I care not how humble it may be, if I find the Bible and a few

well-chosen books upon the shelf, and a
pair of dumb-bells on the floor in the
corner, I always feel that that boy's
future is full of hope and promise. A
pair of dumb-bells weighing but two or
three pounds each cost but a trifle, but
are of great value. If to these can be
added a pair of Indian clubs, an exer-
ciser, and other implements, so much
the better. The exercise can be simple,
but if taken daily, great benefit may confidently be expected.

We have known of boys who desired
to secure an earlier and larger development of the sexual member, and who
sought to secure this result by resorting
to masturbation. Such a course always
proves not only a great sin, but a great
mistake as well. Muscles may be developed by exercise, but by far the most
important part of the sexual member is
the great body of nerves which center
and radiate from the sexual system, in a
series of network which stands related
to the nerves throughout the entire
body. Now instead of being benefited
or strengthened by such a process, these
nerves are impaired, and if this un-

natural act is oft repeated, the nerves are ruined, and thus the mistaken and guilty perpetrator is made to suffer the results of the sin which he has committed in his ignorance.

Not only boys and girls, but men and women as well, need not only to supplement work with exercise, but also need recreation. There is considerable difference between exercise and recreation. Genuine recreation always has in it the element of pleasure. The man who is sawing wood, or breaking stones on the pike, is having exercise, but there is not a sufficient amount of amusement or pleasure in sawing wood or breaking stones, as a continuous daily occupation, to entitle either to be ranked as a recreation. Rolling a hoop, batting a ball, rowing a boat, riding a bicycle, and many other things, have in them a sufficient amount of pleasure for a boy to entitle them to the rank of a recreation. Recreation is always attended with some degree of exercise, but exercise may be, and often is devoid of the element essential to a recreation. The moment therefore that recreation is indulged in to such an extent that it loses the element of exhilaration and pleasure, it then becomes either exercise or toil, according to circumstances. To the child that has been confined for days in the schoolroom or the factory, an hour or two in the park would be a genuine recreation, while to the park police, whose duties demand twelve or fourteen hours each day, the park means work and not recreation.

There are many people, however, who enter into their daily duties with such zest and pleasure that they actually convert their daily duties into a round of perpetual recreation. This truly is the best, as well as the most profitable kind of recreation. You will find boys and girls in the school who take so much pleasure in their studies that, to them, work virtually becomes play. Such boys and girls, and such men and women, are always the healthiest and happiest. They make such a pleasure of business that they do not need to make a business of pleasure. My dear boy, if you want to be healthy, happy, and useful in this world, learn to work, putting yourself into your work with so much earnestness, thoroughness, and enthusiasm that your high and holy purpose shall convert the work into play, or at least that it shall be to you a joy and a delight. Do not make the serious mistake of going out in search of happiness, for then you will never possess it, but do your duty faithfully, and happiness will find you. Happiness can overtake you, but you can never overtake it.

Take your food and your exercise daily. Take recreation as often as you need it, always, however, being sure to choose the best kinds of each. And always remember that even the best may be rendered harmful and injurious by an inappropriate time, an intemperate manner, an undue amount, or by bad associations.

To preserve your health, and secure strength and vigor, you will need also to take plenty of sleep. Eight hours of sleep may be sufficient for many grown people, but for growing boys and girls, ten and twelve out of every twenty-four hours, if taken at the right time, is not more than is needed. Never sit up late, for the earlier hours of the night are by far more valuable for sleep than the late hours. Do not allow yourself to form the habit of lying in bed late in the morning. The old saying may be very common, but it is very, very true, "Early to bed, and early to rise, makes a man healthy, wealthy, and wise." Retire early. Do not sleep on feathers. Go to bed *to* sleep. Don't worry. Keep your conscience clear, and the night will contribute as much to your growth, strength, and vigor as the day.

CYLINDER XVII.

Food and Exercise for the Mind.—The Intellect May Be Starved.—Mind Fed through the Eyes, Ears, and other Senses.—Mental Food Must Be Digested by Thinking, Considering, and other Mental Processes.—Clean Food for the Mind as well as the Body.—The Mental Food Must Be of a Good Quality.—Unwholesome Reading.—Good Reading.—The Spiritual Nature Must also Be Fed.—The Proper Food.—Six Important Rules on Amusements.

MY DEAR FRIEND HARRY: What I said to you last night, and the night before, concerning food, exercise, and recreation for the maintenance of the health of the body, is also true concerning food, exercise, and recreation for the health and development of the mind. The mind needs to be nurtured, or fed, the same as the body. The unused intellectual powers need to be called into exercise, and the mind also needs recreation in the form of amusement. The food for the physical powers enters the body through the mouth, while the food for the brain enters the body through the eyes, ears, and each of the five senses. If you effectually and permanently close the mouth, as in the disease known as lock-jaw, the body will starve, and in like manner, if you close the five entrances or avenues to the brain, the mind will starve. You have seen many people whose bodies were weak and feeble because they did not have a sufficient quantity of nourishing food; and in like manner many people have weak, feeble minds because these people are being starved intellectually. As the body may be starved, not because there is a lack in the quantity, but in the quality of the food, so also with the mind. People may even have food of a good quality, and yet eat it in such a manner, or in such an excessive quantity, that they injure and disease the stomach, and on this account the body starves even while the stomach is full, for you will remember that it is not the quantity which we eat, but the quantity which we digest which nourishes and strengthens.

In the light of these facts you will see,

how important it is that a boy should be taught to become observant and thoughtful concerning all he sees and hears, and also concerning all the sensations conveyed to the mind by means of the five senses. It is not alone what you see and hear that will give strength to your mind and make you intelligent and wise, but what you think upon and inwardly digest that will give strength to your intellectual powers. When you study, think of what you are studying. After reciting your lessons, think of what you have learned. Fully master, or digest, what enters the mind, the same as you digest what enters the stomach, in order that it may become a part of yourself.

Be very careful upon what you feed the mind. As you would not allow dirty food to enter your mouth, so do not allow impurity to be poured into your mind either from books, papers, or the lips of others. Guard your stomach, but guard your mind also.

As you have seen people who were starved and weak because their food was not nourishing, so you and I have seen boys who were great readers; they even neglected important duties in order that they might read, and on the street, in the cars, in the schoolroom they were reading, reading all the time, and yet instead of becoming intelligent, their minds were undisciplined, and they were uninformed and ignorant. The trouble was not that they did not read, but that which they did read was not wholesome reading, and the mind starved and grew weaker from day to day, and year to year.

As I told you in an earlier Talk that you could not injure the body without impairing the mind, so neither can you starve, defile, or injure the mind without injuring the body as well. Read histories and biographies. Read about the sciences and arts. Read of travels and explorations. Read about morals and religion, but do not read stories and trash. The world is too full of good books, and there are too many things in the realm of the actual and the real, concerning which you cannot afford to be ignorant, to permit of the reading of worthless books.

As you have an intelligent nature which must be fed, so you have a moral and spiritual nature which must be fed. As the body, when in health, hungers for food, and the mind for knowledge, so a healthy spiritual nature reaches out after God and after spiritual truths, and if you were to deny yourself the Christian influences of your home, of the Sunday-school, the Church, the Bible, good religious books, and the companionship of Christian people, your spiritual nature would be starved, become weak and unworthy of one whom God has created in His own likeness and in His own image. Feed your physical nature, but feed your intellectual and moral natures also.

As amusements bear to the mind somewhat the same relation that recreation bears to the body, it is proper that I should speak of it here. There are many forms of amusement. Some are unobjectionable, some questionable, and many positively bad. I cannot now particularize, but can state safe principles for government in such matters.

First. Never engage in any amuse-

ment that imposes upon you an extrava-
gant outlay of money. Amusement is a
mere diversion, and to be good it must
not call for a large outlay of anything so
valuable.

Second. It should be of such a character as to furnish the very diversion
and relaxation which your condition
demands—it should not be engaged in
simply for fun.

Third. Your amusement should not
interfere with the rights of others, or put
a cause of stumbling in their path.

Fourth. The amusement which becomes so fascinating that those who
engage in it neglect family or religious
duties, or business obligations, is a
dangerous amusement and should be
avoided.

Fifth. Any amusement which sends
those who engage in it to their duties
the next day with a distaste for the ordinary duties of life, that turns the thought
of the apprentice boy from the tools because they are not swords; the smithy's
boy from his leather apron because it is
not a prince's cloak; and the herdsman
from his cattle because they are not in-

furiated beasts or fighting bulls of the arena is harmful and wholly injurious.

Sixth. The amusement which casts a reproach upon virtue, that suggests doubt about religion or sacred things, that would make you think less of your home, that arrays vice in attractive robes, arouses passion, or benumbs the moral sense is a dangerous amusement and is to be avoided.

In the matter of amusements be thoughtful, conscientious, and careful.

As work may be engaged in with such zest and pleasure as to convert daily toil into perpetual recreation, so study, reading, and mental effort may be entered upon with such enthusiasm and pleasure as to carry into all mental employment and effort that very element which makes amusement attractive and beneficial.

If we bring the right mind and temper to our work, neither recreation nor amusement will afford us any undue temptation or expose us to serious danger.

PART V.

Our Duty to Aid Others to Avoid Pernicious
Habits and to Retain or Regain their Purity and
Strength.

CYLINDER XVIII.

The Superior Surroundings of Some.—Larger
Blessings Mean Larger Responsibilities.—
Our Duty to Those Who Are Less Favorably
Situated.—Duty of the Rescued to Those
Still in Danger.—Many Sin Because Never
Warned.—Those Who Are Neglected Will
Become Enemies to Themselves, to Society,
and to the State.—Bad Boys are Active ;
Why Should Not Good Boys be Active Also?—
Ways of Approach Open to Boys.—Saved
Before They Sin.—Serving the Suffering, or
Saving from Suffering.—Remove Danger
from the Paths of Others.

MY DEAR FRIEND HARRY: After what
I have said in these Talks I am sure that
such an intelligent boy as I have taken
you to be will be grateful for the kind
Providence which gave you being and
place in a home where kind and wise
parents have guarded you from the evils
and sad consequences which pollute and
degrade the lives of so many boys. You
should therefore remember that wherein
we are better than others is due not to

ourselves, but to our kind heavenly
Father, who has placed us where influences and friends have helped us to become better than some others. If they
had enjoyed our privileges and advantages perhaps they would be all that we
are. And may it not also be true that
if we had been born in the midst of the
influences which have surrounded them,
possibly we would be quite like they are?
But do you not know that the advantages and blessings which you have enjoyed place you under obligations to
other boys who are ignorant or sinful,
and who must suffer the sad consequences of their ignorance and vice
unless you and I try to do for them what
others have done for us. Do you not
see that if you had been sleeping in the
midst of enemies who have plotted to
injure and destroy you, and some kind
friend had defeated their purpose and
saved you by awakening you out of
sleep, that when you look and see the
enemies and the injuries which you have
escaped, and then find that others can
only be saved from what you have escaped if someone shall also arouse and

awaken them, do you not see that both
your gratitude and duty demand that you
should do for others what kind friends
have done for you? Manifestly it is our
duty to awaken, warn, and save all who
are exposed to pollution and sin, and to
do all we can to rescue and save the
vicious. Many sin in these matters simply because no one has warned them of
the evil consequences of such a course.

The future condition of multitudes of
boys depends upon what shall be done
for them in these matters. If they are
warned and made intelligent they will
become honorable and useful citizens.
But if no one cares to save them, bad
men and bad boys will exert over them
such influences as will make them enemies to themselves, to society at large,
and to the state and nation. If they are
to be saved they must be saved while
they are young and before habits of vice
have become fixed. They must be helped
to see that vice in any form is an enemy
to their own happiness and well-being,
and be made to feel that the practice is
hateful in the eyes of pure and good
people and sinful in the sight of God.

Bad boys and men are active in their efforts to lead others astray. They lose no opportunity to scatter evil thoughts and vicious practices, and why should not you and all good people seek to spread such useful and helpful information as will assist to save others from sin, from physical and mental weakness, and perhaps from utter ruin.

Boys find ways of approaching other boys upon this subject which are not open to older persons. Being yourself a boy you can approach other boys upon this subject, and especially when subjects of this kind are first mentioned or alluded to by them. If you can save a single boy from sin and vice you will have done a good work. To rescue one who has already gone wrong is to do a good service, but do you not see that to have saved that individual from even beginning such wicked and hurtful practices would be very much better? It is very much as if I should go to the home of a poor man and minister to him day and night for weeks while he was suffering great bodily pain because of broken bones or injuries received from a fall caused by stepping upon a banana skin which some thoughtless person had thrown upon the pavement. If I were thus to care for him in his suffering and distress I would surely be doing a good service. But do you not see that I would be doing a service that is much easier for me and far more beneficial to my poor neighbor if, when I passed down the street just ahead of him, I had shoved the banana skin from the pavement and, with a single little effort, removed from his way the possibility of falling? The work of saving him from falling would be both easier and grander than anything I could do in ministry and service after he had suffered the injury which a little forethought on my part might have prevented.

So you may seek to remove evil and danger from the paths of other boys, and especially from those younger than yourself. Never expose a boy to ridicule lest you break down that sense of shame which must prove helpful to him when he would reform and amend, and lest, being exasperated, he should become reckless and defiant to all sense of modesty and shame. Recommend such boys to read books that will be helpful to them, such as " Kapff's Admonitions " [1]; " Almost a Man," [2] by Dr. Mary Wood-Allen; " Confidential Talks with Young Men," [3] by Dr. Lyman B. Sperry.

In order that you may be intelligent upon this subject and be qualified to suggest and advise others to whom you may come with helpful sympathy, before concluding these Talks I desire to-morrow night to suggest to you some of the most helpful things to be done by those who would make an effort to regain, as far as possible, what they have lost through their ignorance or willful sin in these matters. And then I must bring these Talks to a close by telling something of the changes which you must expect in your own body in the course of a few years, and thus prepare you for experiences and guard you against dangers that lie in your path further on.

[1] A 50-cent book.   [2] A 25-cent booklet.

[3] A 75-cent book. All may be had direct from the Vir Publishing Company, 1134 Real Estate Trust Building, Philadelphia, Pa.

PART VI.

How Purity and Strength May Be Measurably Regained.

CYLINDER XIX.

Purity and Strength, How Regained.—Perfection of Cure Dependent upon the Extent of the Hurt and Method of the Cure.—The Erring Have Much to Hope for.—Human Effort and Divine Help. — Importance of Rules already Suggested. — Months and Years Needed.—Importance of the Bath.— Consult Parents and Competent Physician.— Unnatural Modesty in These Matters.—All Parts to be Held in Purity of Thought.—Important Suggestions Concerning Exercise, Sleep, Diet, etc.—Seek Daily Help from God.

MY DEAR FRIEND HARRY: In harmony with my promise I desire to-night to tell you how purity and strength may be measurably regained by those who have learned the vicious habit which is so prevalent among boys. How fully a boy who has practiced self-pollution may regain his full vigor will depend upon the extent to which he has become addicted to the practice. I think I may best illustrate by saying that

the results will be quite like it is when
one has received a hurt or injury on the
hand or any other portion of the body.
In most instances the hurt may be
healed, but the perfection of the cure
will be dependent upon the extent of the
injury and the wisdom displayed in effecting the cure. No portion of the body
which has suffered an injury can ever
after become absolutely what it was before the hurt, for even when the finger
is simply cut by a sharp blade the cut
may be healed in a few days, but for
years and perhaps for life the individual
must carry the scar which remains after
the wound is healed; and the size of the
scar will depend upon the extent of the
hurt or injury.

Much as the sin is to be regretted and
deplored, yet when a boy awakens to
the importance of a sincere and permanent reformation he is to be encouraged
to hope for and to expect most grati-
fying results if he will but go to God
and confess his sin, seek God's pardon
for the past, accept of Christ as his
Saviour and Helper, and trust Him fully
in his struggle to overcome both his sin

and its consequences. Great results may be expected if the individual co-operates and works with God in this matter. But if human purpose and effort are wanting God will be prevented from doing what He would. Neither God nor man can successfully work alone in such matters. The human effort and the divine help must go together.

All that I said to you a few nights ago, concerning how boys may preserve their entire bodies in purity and strength, is of great importance to boys who would escape from sin and endeavor to regain what they have lost. Carefully recall what I said to you on Cylinders numbered fourteen, fifteen, sixteen, and seventeen. In order that the impression made upon the mind by what I told you then may be deepened, place these cylinders upon the phonograph again and, after listening to them, write down what I said in reference to purity of heart and mind, cleanliness of the body, without and within, the character of all that we put into our bodies in the form of food and drink, the importance of avoiding stimulants of all kinds, the necessity of work, the value of exercise, recreation, amusement, and sleep, and the necessity also for suitable food for the intellectual and moral natures. Everything spoken of on these cylinders is very important to one who desires to become strong and to retain or regain full mastery over self. Emphasizing everything said on these cylinders, there are some directions which need to be somewhat enlarged upon to one who desires to escape from this evil habit and regain what has been lost.

What one seeks who is in this condition, and what is worth all it will cost, cannot be secured in a week, or a month, or even in an entire year. The matter of the largest and best physical development is the result of years of careful and persistent physical culture. The bath is of first importance. To the regular weekly bath should by all means be added the daily morning hand bath in cold water, and if the sexual parts are feverish or sensitive, good results may be secured by adding to these a local bathing of the parts in cold water before retiring in the evening. By placing the bowl upon the floor and crouching over it in a sitting posture, the bath may be most successfully administered. Only in the summer can baths in cold water, in the morning and evening, be begun without the need of great caution to prevent taking cold. But after the body is once accustomed to the application of cold water, the bath itself will fortify the system against taking cold by ordinary exposure.

Where the glans, or end of the sexual member, is sensitive and difficulty is experienced in keeping it clean, or in subduing the irritation, the boy should seek the advice of his parents, who should consult a judicious Christian physician who will be competent to give the boy the sympathy, counsel, and treatment which his particular case may demand. In many cases of this kind, circumcision, which is a very simple surgical operation, is the only effective and permanent cure for the difficulty.

As a boy would go to his parents if he had hurt himself by any misfortune or was suffering from a fever, so he should go to them when injury or sickness attacks him in his sexual members. The feeling which restrains most boys at such times is an unnatural modesty, or is the result of evil practices or vicious thinking. There is no reason why we may not properly speak of this portion of our bodies as of any other portion. Let us remember that God made all parts of our bodies and that all parts are alike sacred. Neither these members themselves nor references to them are unclean or improper until the individual makes them so by his own acts. Every boy who has kind parents owes it to them, to his own present comfort and future happiness and usefulness, that his parents and family physician should be immediately informed of any sickness or infirmity which may afflict him.

If I were speaking to a boy who was desirous of escaping from this vice, in addition to what I have said to you during the previous evenings I would say to him: Take plenty of exercise in the open air. This should be done systematically and regularly; not a little now and then, but daily, and for a sufficient length of time to produce some sense of weariness. Engage the mind also. Avoid all stories and trashy books and papers, but read plenty of good ones. Compel the mind to be attentive. At the end of each page or paragraph stop and recall what you have just been reading about. When you reach the end, turn back and review each chapter. Discipline both your body and your mind. Teach both body and mind to obey the will. This is very important, for the effort develops character, genders strength, and makes a boy masterly and masterful.

Sleep on a hard bed in a properly ventilated room. Let the covers be slightly deficient, rather than overmuch. Do not sleep on your back. Avoid feather beds, either to lie upon or as a covering, except in the most extreme climate and under the most extreme circumstances. Sleep apart in a bed by yourself. Do not choose cushioned chairs. Avoid horseback riding. Abstain from stimulants in all forms, including tea and coffee; cocoa and chocolate are much to be preferred. To all boys and men suffering from sexual irritation and weakness intoxicating liquors of all kinds, and tobacco in every form, are specially injurious.

Be careful about the diet. Milk and vegetable foods are most favorable to a mastery of sexual sensitiveness, but a moderate quantity of fresh meat should be used to prevent weakness and debility. Fresh fish are good, but eggs should be used with due moderation. Pork is bad; salt meats are difficult to digest, and are not nutritious. Pepper, pickles, and condiments are to be avoided. Pies and cakes disorder the stomach and result in injury on that account. Candy, if it be eaten at all, should be eaten in moderation and not beween meals. Be careful that the trousers are not made to press too tightly against the sexual organs because of suspenders that are too short. Shun sinful companions. Turn from evil pictures. Avoid the temptations which are occasioned by being much alone. Seek the companionship of the good. Aspire to some high and holy purpose in life; ask God's help daily, and press forward, regaining depleted powers; be daunted by no difficulties, persevere, and God will help, and the victory and blessing which await will be yours.

This, my dear boy, would be my advice to any boy who would turn his back upon the wicked past and turn his face hopefully to the future.

PART VII.

The Age of Puberty, and its Attendant Changes.

CYLINDER XX.

The Passage from Infancy to Manhood.—
Physical and Mental Changes that Occur at
the Age of Puberty.—Meaning of the Term
" Puberty." — The Dormant or Sleeping
Powers.—They Awake and Fully Mature by
the Time We Need Them.—From Fourteen
to Twenty-five the Man is Maturing.—Prior
to Puberty Boys and Girls Much Alike in
Characteristics.—At Fourteen the Manly
Characteristics Begin to Develop. — The
New and Embarrassing Experiences.—The
Divinely Implanted Nature Awakes.—The
Attendant Dangers. — How the Boy Is
Affected.—It Is the Period of "Storm and
Stress."—Dangers which Arise from Igno-
rance.—Importance of Intelligence.

MY DEAR FRIEND HARRY: Not many
years ago the cradle in which your baby
sister sleeps was yours. But to-day you
have passed on beyond the cradle and
are pressing forward toward manhood
and a life of usefulness, honor, and blessing. For just a few years you will continue to be a boy, and then, at about the

age of fourteen or fifteen, you will enter
upon a period of several years during
which time those portions of the reproductive system which are hidden away
in the interior and lower portions of your
body will begin to develop, and you
will experience emotions which indicate
changes that will be altogether new
and strange. The physical and mental
changes that occur at that time, and the
conditions which attend them, to many
boys prove a time of great mystery, perplexity, and danger. That this chang-
ing condition may not come upon you
unawares, but that you may meet it with
intelligent understanding, I desire to tell
you in advance something concerning
that period in the life of every boy which
is called "the age of puberty." In
speaking of plants, the word "puberty"
means the period when the plant first
begins to bear flowers. In boys it is the
period in which the reproductive or
sexual organs begin to develop and
sexual fluid first begins to form in the
glands situated in the interior and lower
portion of the body.

When we are born into the world as

helpless infants, God does not immediately give us all the powers and endowments which we shall need later on, but for which we at that time have no use. But these powers He gives us as we have need of them. At first the baby has no need of teeth, but after a year or two God gives it a few, and then adds others, from time to time, as there is necessity. When the child is born the beginnings of the teeth are hidden under the gums. They are in embryo, as learned men say, awaiting the appointed time to grow, when the child is older and has use for them. In this same way the reproductive system in all healthy children remains undeveloped, in embryo, dormant, or sleeping until the age of about fourteen or fifteen, when this system begins to awake and grow, and various changes begin to take place which are gradually, through a period of years, to lift and change the boy from a child into the fully developed man.

These changes, which take place between the age of fourteen and twenty-five, but which are most marked and most trying between the ages of fourteen and eighteen, are very important, and, as many in their ignorance and lack of knowledge fall into vice and sin and come to early or eventual ruin, it is important that all boys should know what to expect, so that they may interpret to themselves the true meaning of their new experiences and trying conditions.

The greatest outward or visible changes take place rapidly, requiring but a year or two to effect very noticeable results. But the most critical period, during which the greatest internal and invisible, physical and mental changes are taking place is, at least in most instances, from fourteen to twenty-one, but the changes are not fully completed and full sexual maturity attained until the age of about twenty-five.

During the earlier years of life, while the reproductive organs are dormant and undeveloped, boys and girls are much alike in most of their physical and mental traits. But at about the age of fourteen—with some earlier and with others later—as they approach the period of puberty, the characteristics and traits peculiar to the sex begin to develop, the boys becoming more manly and the girls becoming more womanly.

When this time arrives the boy begins to leave behind him the characteristics of childhood. The body grows rapidly. The shoulders become broader, the chest deeper. The voice loses its boyish tones and becomes deeper and stronger. The skin becomes coarser. The beard starts to grow. The bones become harder. The sexual parts begin to develop, and in a few years the wisdom teeth appear.

At first the boy feels awkward. His voice breaks. His hands and his feet seem to be in his way. He is sensitive and bashful under circumstances where formerly he was at ease and at home. He becomes the subject of new sensations and new desires, which he is not able to interpret or to comprehend. He becomes more polite, and more manly in his bearing toward strangers, and especially toward women. He begins to seek the companionship of girls of about his own age. All this time there is being awakened and quickened within him a divinely implanted nature, which is designed to make him more noble and more perfect in every respect than he could possibly be without it.

But it is now that sexual passion begins to assert itself. If the boy is ignorant, has a weak moral sense, or is under the influence of evil companions, serious dangers are likely to follow. It is also at this critical time, between the ages of thirteen and twenty-one, that boys become irritable and petulant. They experience a feeling of contrariness. They are untractable and at times even rebellious. It is during this period that many boys and girls, whose parents do not understand their condition, and who have forgotten their own feelings and experiences when at the same age, desire to break loose from all restraint and sometimes even to run away from home. It is at this time that the boy who was formerly obedient and studious often becomes restive, disobedient, and unruly. Boys between the years of fourteen and eighteen are more likely to be disobedient to their teachers in the day school, and it is just at this age that they are likely to feel that they are too old

to go to Sunday-school, and are not so
likely to go willingly to church or attend
to their religious duties. The entire
nature feels the revolution that is taking
place, and all the worst qualities in the
boy's composition appear upon the surface. This is the period in the boy's
experience which the Germans call " The
period of storm and stress." If the boy
is made intelligent, and his parents and
teachers understand and appreciate what
the boy is passing through, all will
eventually turn out better than the indi-
cations seem to promise, and as the
young man approaches the age of twenty
and upward the storm will have passed
by. And if he has been guarded from
evil and kept from sin his future will be
increasingly calm, blessed, and prosper-
ous. But if vice and evil have come into
his life the years will bring an increasing
installment of passion and sin, of disappointment and suffering.

You see, my dear boy, how important
it is that at this time, which is usually
the most trying in one's entire life, that
a boy should not be left to grope in darkness and ignorance among physical and

moral dangers of the most serious nature. Only those who have passed through this "time of storm and stress," and have been observant of their emotions and experiences, and have thought and reasoned intelligently concerning them, can wholly appreciate the keen, sensitive condition, the strong temptations, and the great need of wise counsel, helpful sympathy, and the assistance of some-one who will know how to interpret to the inexperienced the lessons which God is teaching and the great duties and re-sponsibilities for which God, in infinite wisdom and love, is preparing the com-ing man.

To-morrow night I will send you my last cylinder, and I shall desire to advise you how to prepare for this approaching change and make a few other sugges-tions which are prompted by my love for you and my abounding interest in boys and young men.

CYLINDER XXI.

The Last Talk.—Desire to Prepare You for the Coming Manhood.—Purity like the Dew.—Boys Impatient for Developing Manhood.—Different Ages at which Puberty Occurs in Different Individuals. — Causes of Diversity.—Appears Earliest in Diseased Bodies and Latest in the Healthiest.—Illustrated in Diseased Fruit.—The Boys with the Best Bodily Health Experience the Least Trials during the Developing Years.—Early Development Means Early Decay.—Years of Adolescence a Period of Special Danger.—Our Parting Counsel.—Danger of Deferring.—Immediate Development of Physical, Intellectual, and Moral Powers of Utmost Importance.—"How Shall We Escape if We Neglect."—Moral Nature Most Important of All.—What Satan Will Say.—The Results Are Inevitable.—Do Not Defer.—Covenant with God.

My Dear Friend Harry: Nearly a month has passed since I began these Talks to you into the phonograph. I have spoken to you out of a heart full of interest and sympathy for boys, and what otherwise would have been a task has been to me a source of no little pleasure. I am to-night to have my last Talk with you upon these important subjects, and I am pleased to hope that all I have said from night to night has been to you a matter of valuable interest and satisfactory information.

By what I said last night you will see that I have desired to prepare your mind for the changes which you must meet a little later on in life. I have desired that in your passage from boyhood to manhood you may avoid the perplexities and dangers which prove so disastrous to many. Purity is something like the dew which in the morning sparkles in ·crystal beauty on grass and flower, but when once brushed away by a ruthless hand it cannot be restored by art or skill of man, although all the waters of the world were placed at his command.

Knowing how natural it is for all boys to desire to be men, and how impatient some boys become when they note in others developments and changes which have not come to them, I desire to apprise you of a serious mistake in judgment which most boys make, and which is liable to prompt them to evil practices. These practices, instead of hastening manly development, result in weakness and disease, and, as a consequence, defeat the very end they have sought to secure.

The age at which puberty is reached, and the changes take place, concerning which I told you last night, varies in different individuals. In boys these changes begin in rare and exceptional cases as early as twelve years, while in other exceptional cases they are delayed as late as the eighteenth year. This variation is due somewhat to nationality, race, or, more frequently, to climate, but most frequently to conditions of bodily disease or health in the individual. In warm countries this development comes earlier, and in the cold northwest climate, much later. Colored boys tend to develop earlier than white boys. Temperament, occupation, and habits have much to do in determining this matter, but, as I said, the condition of the health produces the greatest variation of all. It is generally found that boys who have inherited a weak, nervous constitution, or who suffer from poor health, are the first to develop the changes which indicate the approach and presence of puberty; while, upon the other hand, the general rule is that the boys who live mostly in the open air, are engaged in pursuits which call for vigorous bodily exercise, and who are given to such manly sports as develop a strong body and good health, are slower in experiencing these changes.

This is only another manifestation of what every boy has noticed in fruit. While growing upon the trees the first few apples, peaches, cherries, and other kinds of fruit that turn red and appear ripe, while the great mass of fruit has not yet approached maturity, may look promising to the eye, but when they are examined they are always found to be wormy and diseased.

The boy who seeks early maturity by sinful practices only secures in its place weakness and disease, while the boy who is careful to observe all the laws of health, and who develops a strong, manly frame, and establishes good bodily health, will experience less irritation, nervousness, and sexual sensitiveness, and will pass into manhood without encountering the trials and perplexities which come to those who suffer from inherited or acquired bodily weakness or disease. By no means, my dear boy, ever covet that early development which could confer upon you nothing that is to be truly desired, for early maturity means early decay.

By proper food, daily bathing, and by exercise in the fresh air, which should not be too violent nor too prolonged, but yet sufficiently frequent and vigorous, you should seek to acquire that bodily and mental vigor which will prepare you for many years of good health and great usefulness.

The years of adolescence, which begin in boys at about the age of fourteen and continue until they are about twenty-five, are fraught with perplexities, trials, and much danger. It is during these years that most boys make mistakes and go wrong; some physically, some intellectually, some morally, and some in all three of these respects.

These mistakes for the most part grow out of the ignorance of the individual. I am persuaded that very few boys deliberately and willfully go wrong, but they sin in their ignorance, and continue until vices become fixed habits, and ruin becomes inevitable.

It is on this account that I have thought it necessary to apprise you of these changes, that being warned in early boyhood you may, by physical culture, acquire such bodily strength and vigor as will enable you to pass through this period with perfect safety, and enter upon your mature years a noble, pure, and godly man. If you will remember what I have said, and be faithful to carry out the suggestions which I have made, I think you will be in possession of such information upon the subject of the reproductive organs as will serve you until your fifteenth or sixteenth year, when you will need the further information and suggestions which I have embodied in a book entitled "What a Young Man Ought to Know," and which I was just completing when I received your Mamma's note, which led to my sending you the series of Talks in the phonograph which will be concluded with this cylinder.

And now, my dear friend Harry, before parting, I desire to warn you against one dangerous mistake which thousands of people make—namely, the mistake of deferring. You may admit the truth of all that I have said, and honestly purpose to accept and act upon it, but instead of doing so immediately you may defer to some future time, and thus by neglect eventually and irretrievably lose all that you hope to attain. You may reason, as so many do, that you are strong and well; that you are reasonably happy; and that, as you are still very young, you can indulge your appetite, neglect your soul, violate God's physical and moral laws, and later on, atone for the past by proper exercise, careful diet, and a religious life. While you have been saved from the secret sin which is ruining others, yet the care of your health, and the development of your physical, intellectual, and spiritual powers, are of the utmost immediate importance. At no other time in your life can you so easily

and successfully acquire the best of each
of these desirable endowments as at the
immediate present.

Let the words from the Scriptures ring
in your ears, " HOW SHALL WE ESCAPE IF
WE NEGLECT? " (Hebrews ii. 3.) In
order to grow up in ignorance, all that a
boy needs to do is to neglect his books
and his school. In order to become a
bankrupt, a merchant need not squander
his money; he need not make unprofit-
able investments; simply let him neglect
his business duties, and bankruptcy is
inevitable. The farmer does not need to
sow his fields with weeds. Simply let
him neglect his fields, and weeds will fill
them, thorns and bushes will half conceal
his broken fences, and universal ruin will
come as the inevitable result of simple
neglect.

And so, my dear boy, even though you
have already attained the very best physical, intellectual, and spiritual culture,
yet if you fail to guard and keep such
attainments by constant exercise and use,
you will surely lose them. If these things
are so, then how shall you escape from
the result of indifference and delay, if in

the beginning you neglect these important matters?

You may accept and act upon what I
have suggested concerning your physical
and intellectual natures but neglect
your spiritual nature, which is most
important of all. Satan is sure to whis-
per that what I have said is all true, but
that you are young, and that later on in
life, after you have finished your school
days, and are established in business,
then you will have plenty of time to attend to spiritual matters, and thus tempt
you, from year to year, simply to defer
until your best years, and if possible,
all your years, shall have been lost to
Christ and your own happiness by simple
neglect.

No; do not defer, do not neglect. For
if you do, you cannot escape from the sad
results of such a mistake. Weakness
and disease will then be sure to despoil
you of manly power; ignorance will set
up its throne where intelligence should
reign, and the spiritual nature, which
God would restore again to His own
likeness and image, Satan will further
disfigure and deface by vice and sin.

These results are inevitable, and cannot be escaped if you neglect.

My dear boy, do not defer. May I ask you now, as I bid you good-by to-night, to go apart immediately, and alone upon your knees ask God, for Christ's sake, to forgive your sins, to give you a clean, pure, and loving heart, and to take you into everlasting covenant with Himself. Covenant to serve Him faithfully from this hour, and may God abundantly bless you in this world, and in the next crown you with everlasting honor and glory!

THE END.

OFFICES OF PUBLICATION

IN THE UNITED STATES

THE VIR PUBLISHING COMPANY

2237 LAND TITLE BUILDING
PHILADELHHIA, PA.

IN ENGLAND

THE VIR PUBLISHING COMPANY

7 IMPERIAL ARCADE, LUDGATE CIRCUS
LONDON, E. C.

IN CANADA

WILLIAM BRIGGS

29-33 RICHMOND STREET WEST
TORONTO, ONTARIO

"What a Young Man Ought to Know"

WHAT EMINENT PEOPLE SAY

Francis E. Clark, D. D.

"It is written reverently but very plainly, and I believe will save a multitude of young men from evils unspeakable."

John Clifford, D. D.

"One of the best books for dawning manhood that has fallen into my hands. It goes to the roots of human living. It is thoroughly manly."

J. Wilbur Chapman, D. D.

"I bear willing testimony that I believe this book ought to be in the hands of every young man in this country."

Paul F. Munde, M. D., LL. D.

Professor of Gynæcology in the New York Polyclinic and at Dartmouth College.

"I most heartily commend not only the principle but the execution of what it aims to teach."

The Right Rev. William N. McVickar, D. D.

"I heartily endorse and recommend 'What a Young Man Ought to Know.' I believe that it strikes at the very root of matters."

Ethelbert D. Warfield, LL. D.

"The subject is one of the utmost personal and social importance, and hitherto has not been treated, so far as I am aware, in such a way as to merit the commendation of the Christian public.

Frank W. Ober

"It will save many a young fellow from the blast and blight of a befouled manhood, wrecked by the wretched blunderings of an ignorant youth."

Frederick Anthony Atkins

"Such books as yours have long been needed, and if they had appeared sooner many a social wreck, whose fall was due to ignorance, might have been saved."

"What a Young Girl Ought to Know"

WHAT EMINENT PEOPLE SAY

Francis E. Willard, LL.D.

"I do earnestly hope that this book, founded on a strictly scientific but not forgetting a strong ethical basis, may be well known and widely read by the dear girls in their teens and the young women in their homes."

Mrs. Elizabeth B. Grannis

"These facts ought to be judiciously brought to the intelligence of every child whenever it asks questions concerning its own origin."

Mrs. Harriet Lincoln Coolidge

"It is a book that mothers and daughters ought to own."

Mrs. Katharine L. Stevenson

"The book is strong, direct, pure, as healthy as a breeze from the mountain-top."

Mrs. Isabelle MacDonald Alden, "Pansy"

"It is just the book needed to teach what most people do not know how to teach, being scientific, simple and plain-spoken, yet delicate."

Miss Grace H. Dodge

"I know of no one who writes or speaks on these great subjects with more womanly touch than Mrs. Wood-Allen, nor with deeper reverence. When I listen to her I feel that she has been inspired by a Higher Power."

Ira D. Sankey

"Every mother in the land that has a daughter should secure for her a copy of "What a Young Girl Ought to Know." It will save the world untold sorrow."

⁵⁴ "What a Young Woman Ought to Know"

WHAT EMINENT PEOPLE SAY

Lady Henry Somerset

"An extremely valuable book, and I wish that it may be widely circulated."

Mrs. Laura Ormiston Chant

"The book ought to be in the hands of every girl on her fifteenth birthday, as a safe guide and teacher along the difficult path of womanhood."

Margaret Warner Morley

"There is an awful need for the book, and it does what it has undertaken to do better than anything of the kind I ever read."

Mrs. May Wright Sewall

"I am profoundly grateful that a subject of such information to young woman should be treated in a manner at once so noble and so delicate."

Elizabeth Cady Stanton

"It is a grave mistake for parents to try to keep their children ignorant of the very questions on which they should have scientific information."

Lillian M. N. Stevens

"There is a great need of carefully, delicately written books upon the subjects treated in this series. I am gratefully glad that the author has succeeded so well, and I trust great and enduring good will be the result."

Mrs. Matilda B. Carse

"It is pure and instructive on the delicate subjects that mean so much to our daughters, to their future as homekeepers, wives and mothers, and to the future generations."

"Manhood's Morning"
BY JOSEPH ALFRED CONWELL

An Invaluable Book for Every Young Man

Chapter 1, Twelve Million Young Men. Chapter 2, The Best Years of Life. Chapter 3, What Some Young Men Have Done. Chapter 4, Wild Oats and Other Weeds. Chapter 5, Reason Why Young Men Go Wrong. Chapter 6, Paying the Piper. Chapter 7, Where Young Men Belong. Chapter 8, What Young Men Must Be. Chapter 9, What Young Men Must Do.

COMMENDATIONS

From Prof. Lyman B. Sperry, M.D., Lecturer and Author

"Every young man should read it yearly from the time he is fourteen till he is twenty-eight."

Bishop J. H. Vincent, LL.D., Chancellor of Chautauqua University

"Every minister who deals with young men, and every young man who cares to avoid evil and loves righteousness should read the book."

Frances E. Willard, President National W. C. T. U.

"We advise parents to send for a copy of this book to give as a present to their sons."

T. J. Sanders, A.M., Ph.D., President Otterbein University, Ohio

"A remarkable series of Chapters to young men—stimulating and suggestive."

Price, $\left\{ \begin{array}{c} \$1.00 \\ 4 \text{ s.} \end{array} \right\}$ net, per Copy

Talks to the ❧ King's Children

Second Series of "Five-Minute Object Sermons."

BY

SYLVANUS STALL, D. D.

Invaluable in ⎰ The Home
The Sunday School
The Pastor's Library
The Mission Field

❧

A CHILDREN'S PREACHER.

" Dr. Stall has few equals in this particular line of writing. He shows a fine reserve in not allowing the object used to over-shadow the truth taught."—*Nashville Christian Advocate.*

" The Rev. Dr. Sylvanus Stall is one of the best preachers for young people in the American pulpit. His ' Five-minute Object Sermons' to children was an ideal book in its class. The present volume is a second series of the same kind, and will be found to have no less point and charm than the volume published two years ago."—*New York Independent.*

" The author is well-known in this community, having been a pastor in Baltimore City for several years. He is an adept certainly in furnishing bright, interesting talks to children. He writes with a vigorous, irresistible pen."—*Baltimore Methodist.*

THE CHILDREN GOOD JUDGES.

" Those who have had the genuine pleasure and profit of Dr. Stall's first series of children's sermons will welcome this second volume. We have read them with the children and commend them very highly. The children know a good sermon when they hear it."—*Reformed Church Messenger.*

" Irresistibly interesting, especially to the young mind."— *Christian Work.*

Price, $1.00 per copy.

Five-minute Object Sermons To Children

BY

SYLVANUS STALL, D. D.

"Through Eye-Gate and Ear-Gate into the City of Child-Soul."

PRESS NOTICES

"They are animated in style, bright, interesting, and practical."—*The Advance.*

"The object of the author is to present the cardinal truths of salvation in simple language, illustrated by common every-day objects, after the manner of our Lord's parables. Delightful and instructive reading for the family circle on Sunday afternoons."—*The Ram's Horn.*

"It begins with an introductory essay, which is a capital treatment of the whole question of children in church, and well worth the cost of the book. He never fails in interest and instruction."—*Sunday-School Times.*

"We do not know that we can give a stronger commendation to this little volume than to state that on a brief examination of it we got the suggestion for a series of half a dozen evening sermons to the young people."—*The Christian Statesman.*

"Excellent, admirable, irresistible. The author is a genius. There is not a dull line between these covers. The author exhibits a new way of preaching the Gospel. The deepest truths are presented in the concrete."—*The Golden Rule.*   Price, $1.00 per copy.

Five-minute Object Sermons—Continued

Unsolicited Commendations

12mo, Cloth, 253 pp. Price, $1.00, post free.

ADDRESS ALL ORDERS TO

THE VIR PUBLISHING COMPANY